Nutraville

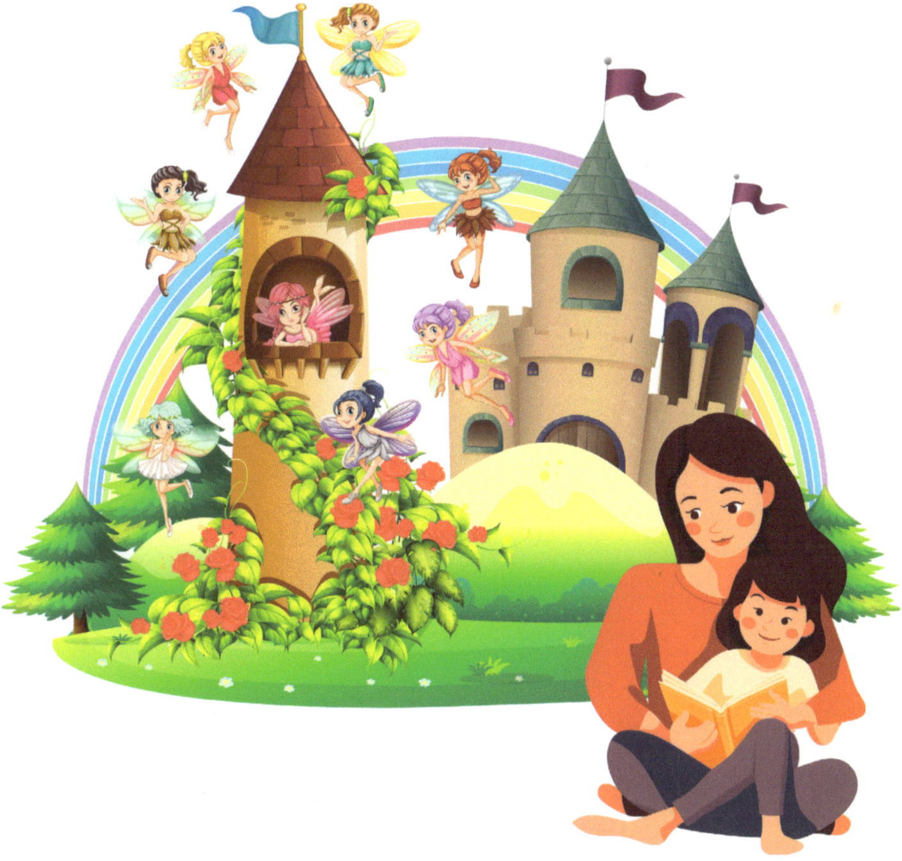

This book is dedicated to :

To all kids of this world, bright and bold,
Your curiosity and hunger for knowledge, like gold.
With nutrition as your guiding star,
Together, let's build a beautiful and healthier world,
near and far.

Hello young adventurers! Welcome to the world of nutrition with Samta, your fearless friend on a mission to uncover the secrets of healthy eating for kids! From battling food allergies to discovering the magic of nourishing food, join me on an exciting journey of delicious discoveries.

Hailing from the mystical Himalayas and now making my home in New Jersey, USA, I'm a mompreneur, fitness coach, and nutritionist dedicated to helping kids like you thrive through nutritious choices. Through my company RTB Kombucha, we brew up tasty probiotic drinks to keep your body and soul happy and healthy.

In my book all about kids' nutrition, you'll learn how to be food superheroes by making smart decisions about what you eat. Let's embark on this fun-filled adventure together and unlock the amazing powers of nutritious foods!

Excited to have you join me on this quest for health and happiness,

-Samta

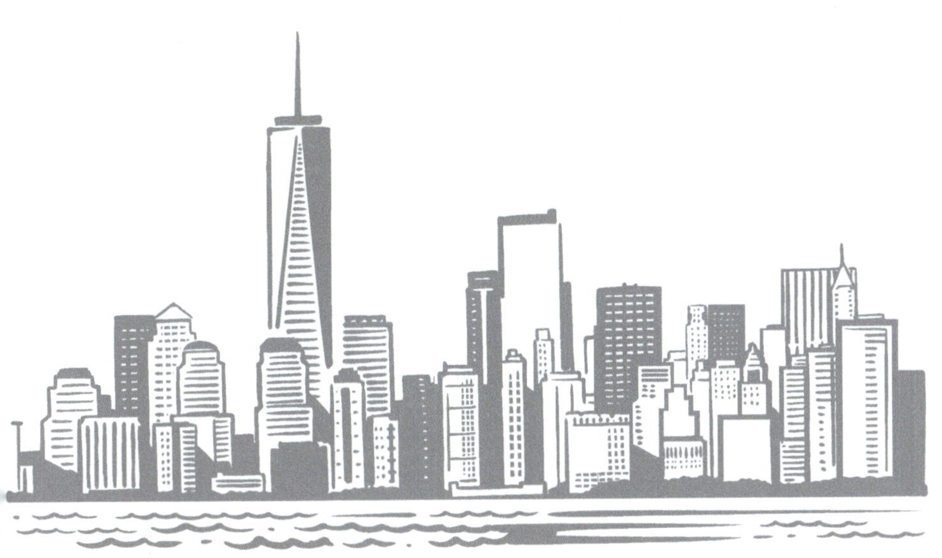

In the busy city of dreams
called New York, there
was a lively girl named
Ruhaani.

She had big dreams and loved life with lots of energy. Ruhaani started dancing and doing gymnastics when she was just three years old because she enjoyed moving and being graceful.

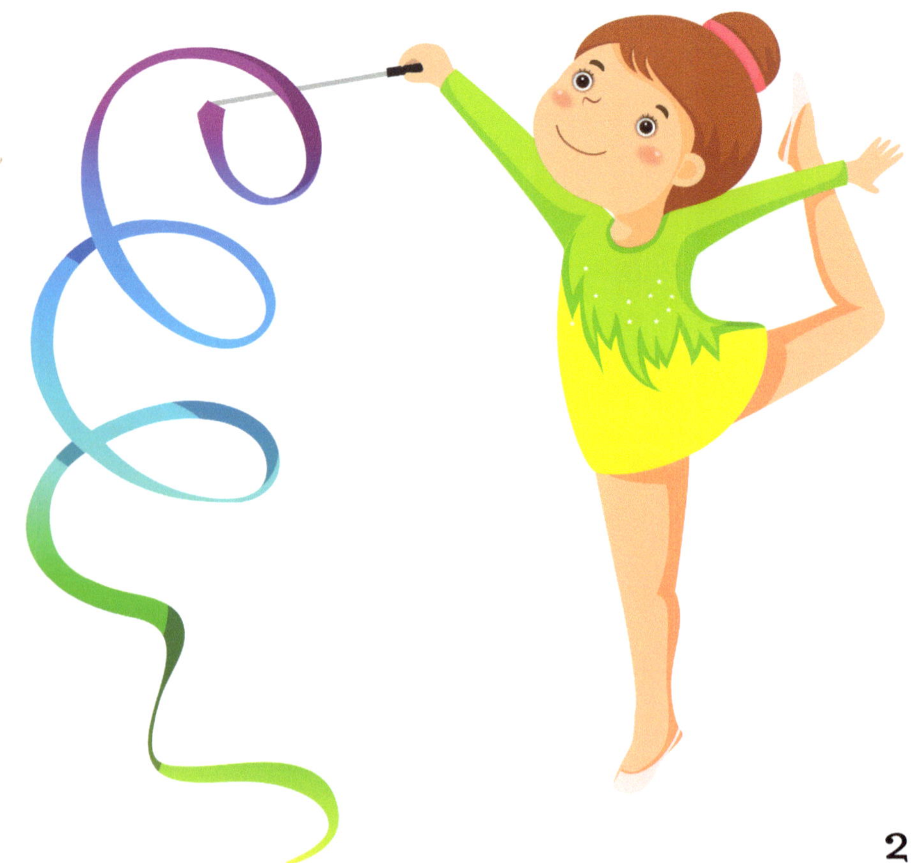

2

She was always moving and trying new things like gymnastics with great enthusiasm.

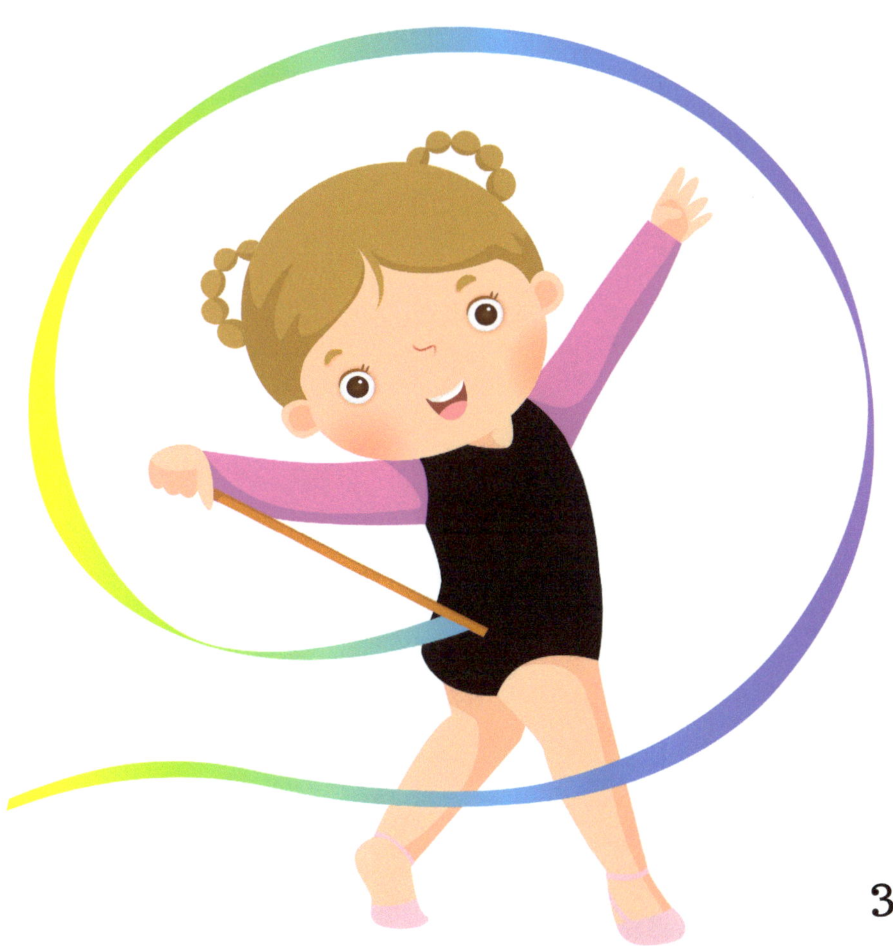

3

However, she started feeling very tired as time went on. Despite her hard work, she struggled to keep up her energy for training and competing.

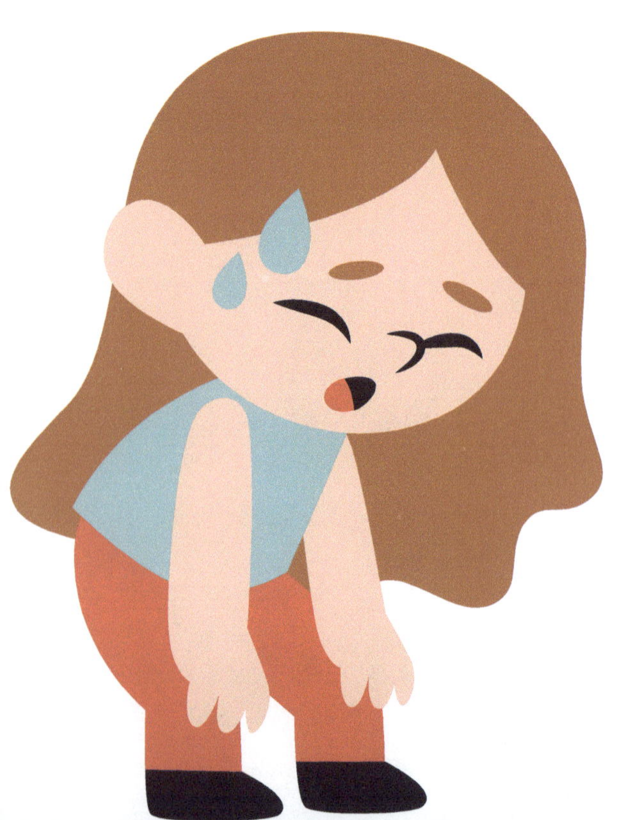

This made her wonder why she was feeling so exhausted. Over time, her worry increased as she felt drained by the constant fatigue.

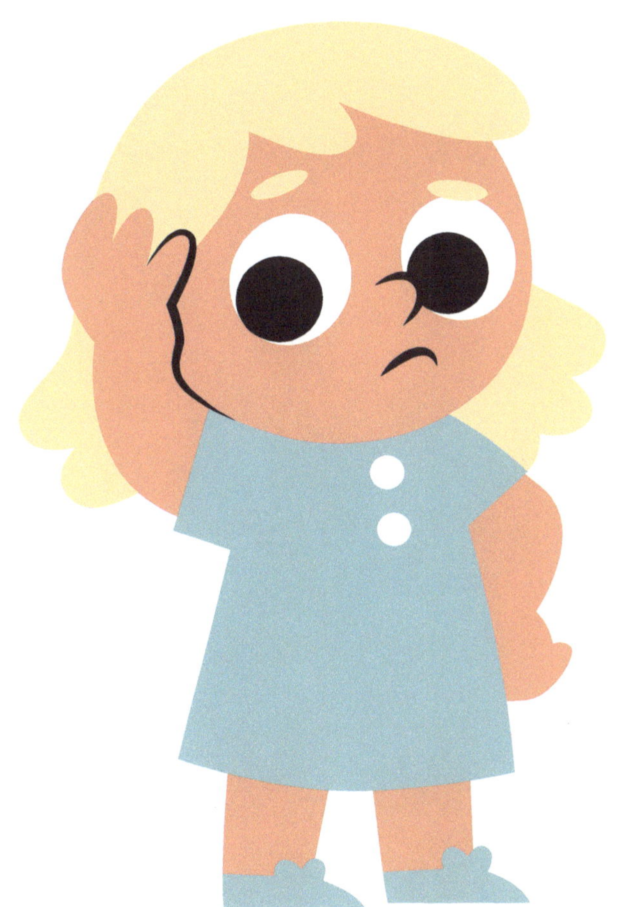

She asked her experienced mother, who is a renowned nutritionist, for advice on how to change her habits.

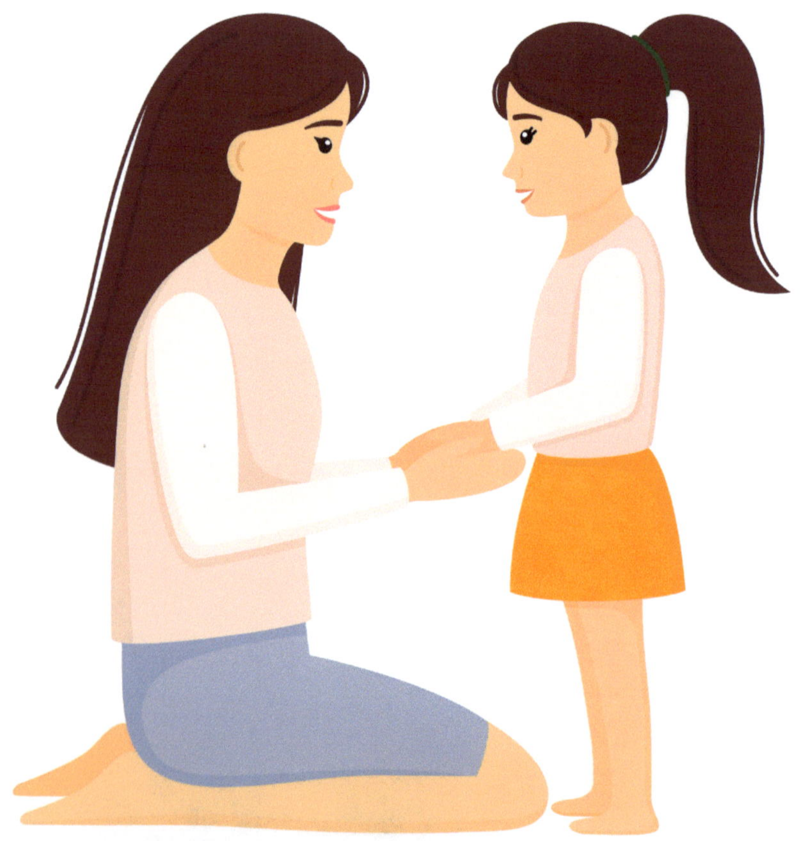

Her mother's wise advice and knowledge gave her comfort when she had doubts. Ruhaani's mother kindly held her hand and guided her on a journey to learn about nutrition and healthy eating. Her mom told an engaging story, and they had a great time pretending together.

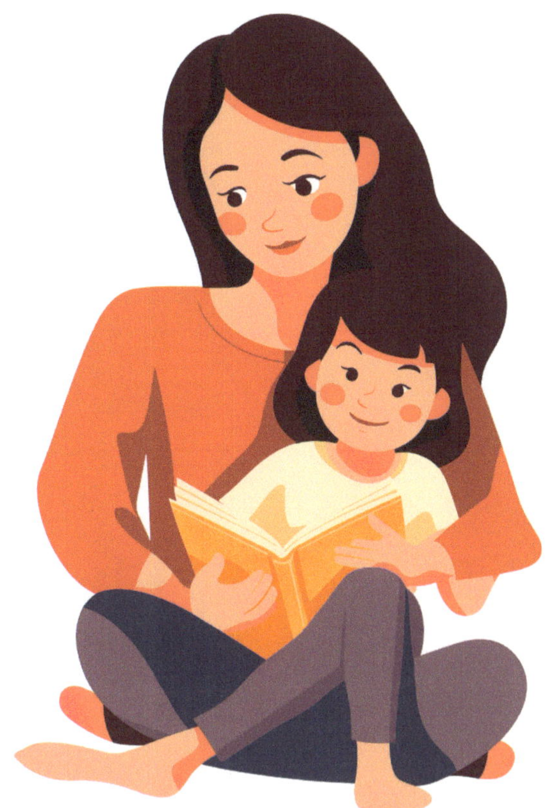

Mom told a story about a girl named Rooh who lived in a place called Nutraville.

Nutraville

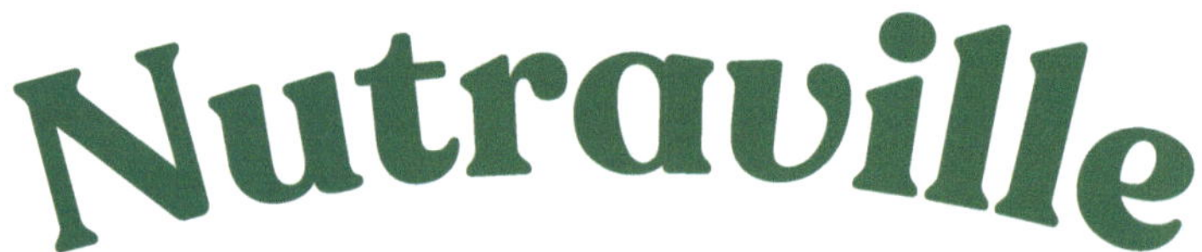

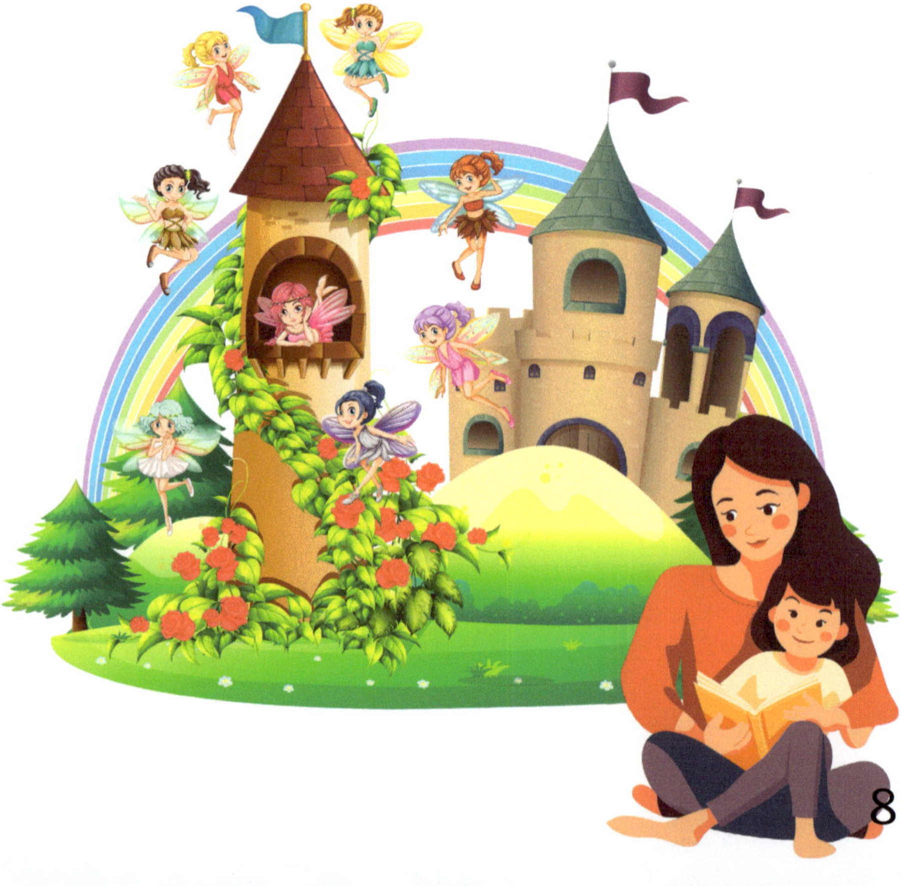

8

Rooh had a special ability to see beyond
the appearance of the food in her
kingdom.
She believed she knew everything
about food, drinks, and how to live a
healthy life.

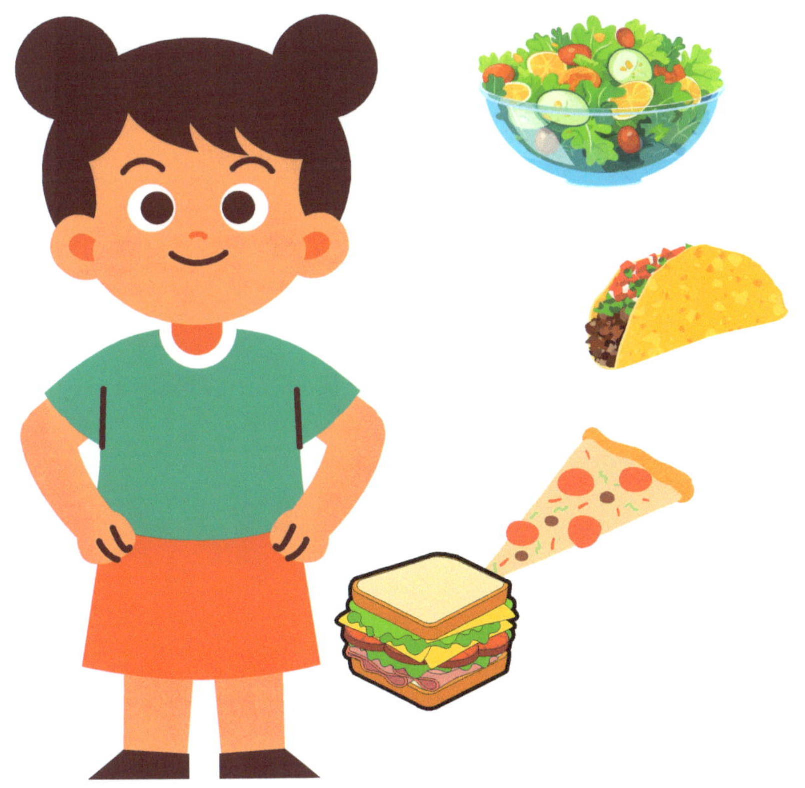

A wise Nutrition Wizard visited Rooh,
who thought she was already eating
healthy
foods.

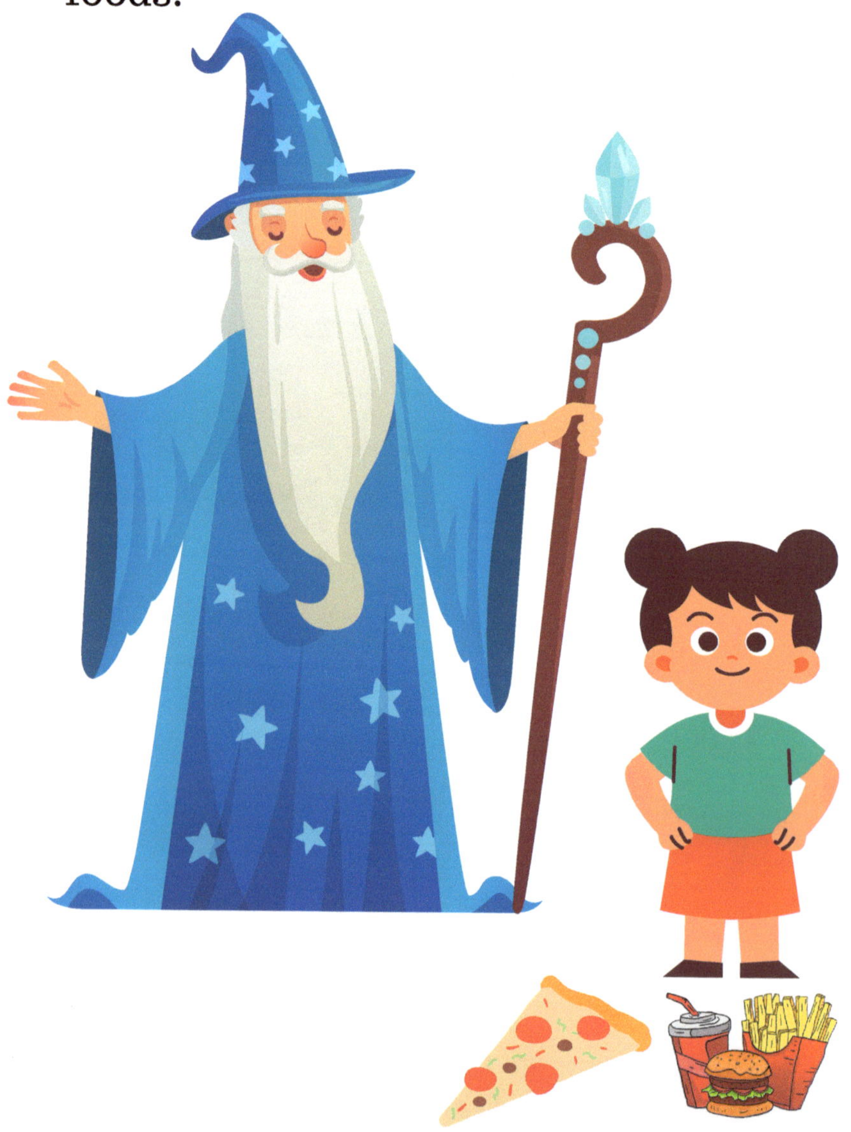

The Nutrition Wizard explained that packaged foods have a Nutrition Label with important information about ingredients and nutrients.

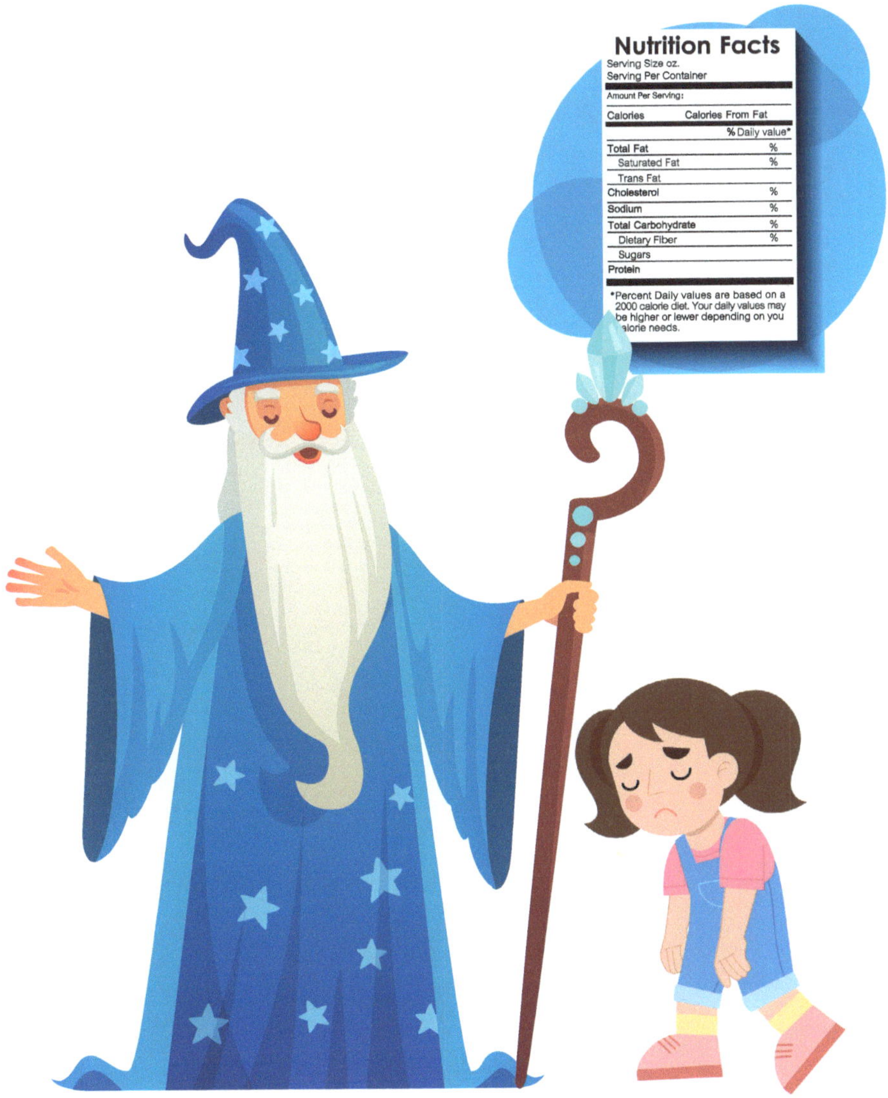

Rooh needed to become a food detective to understand this information hidden in the labels.

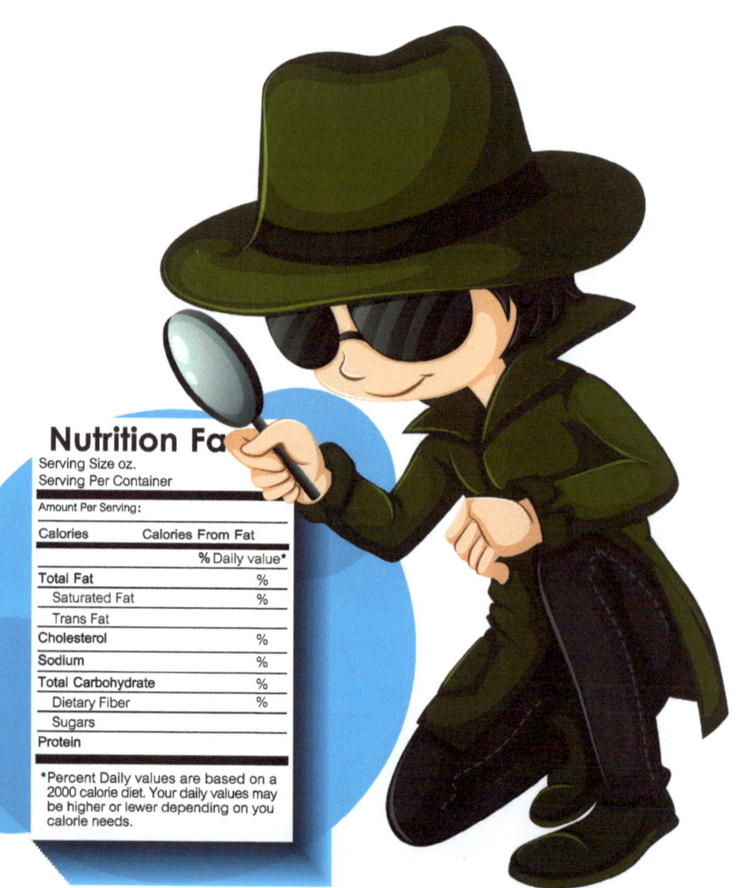

Rooh and the Nutrition Wizard worked together on exciting adventures to understand good, quantified nutrition, Nutrition labels on various foods.

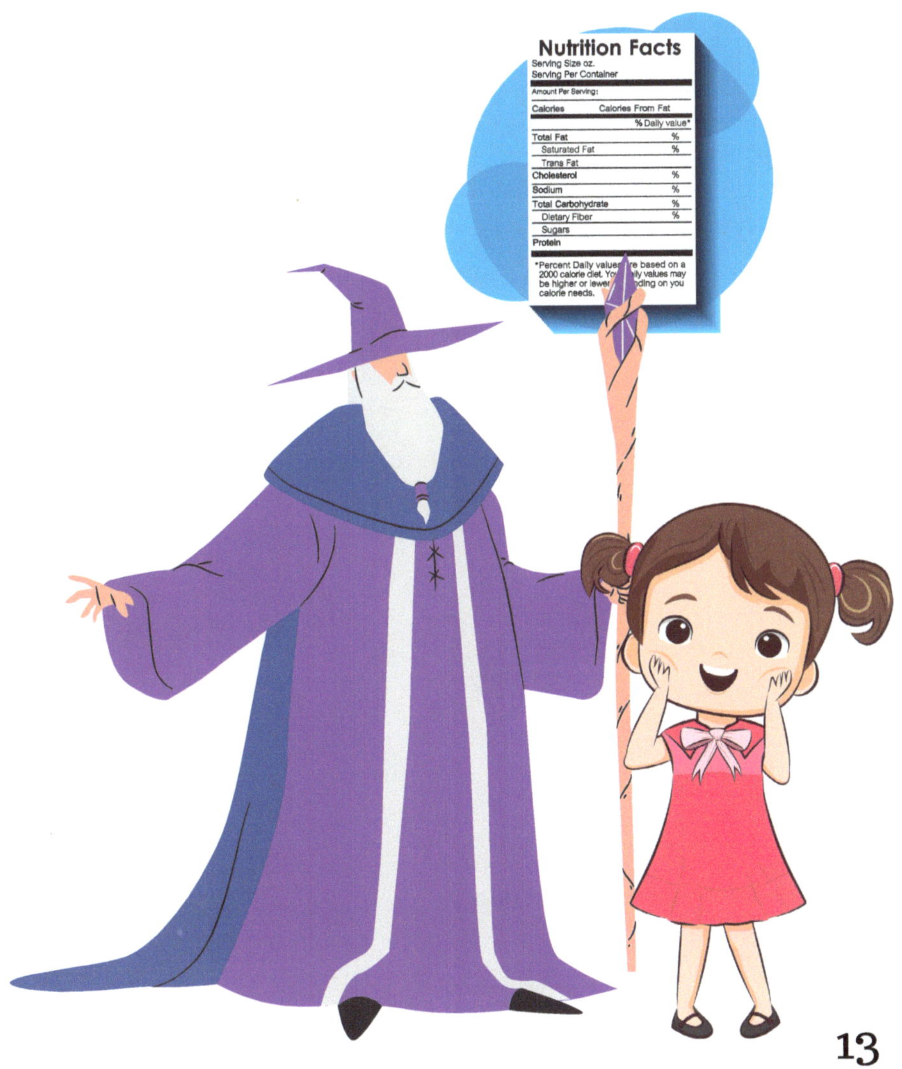

They figured out the secret information and discovered what are macronutrients (Protein, Fat, Carbohydrates) and ...

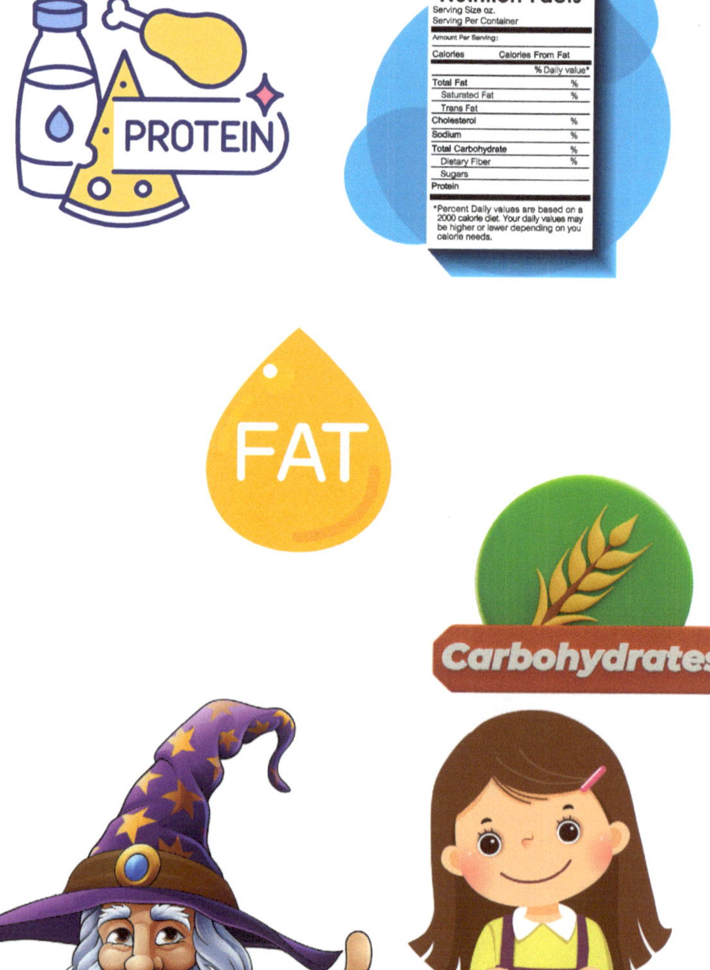

What are micronutrients (minerals, vitamins) in each product.

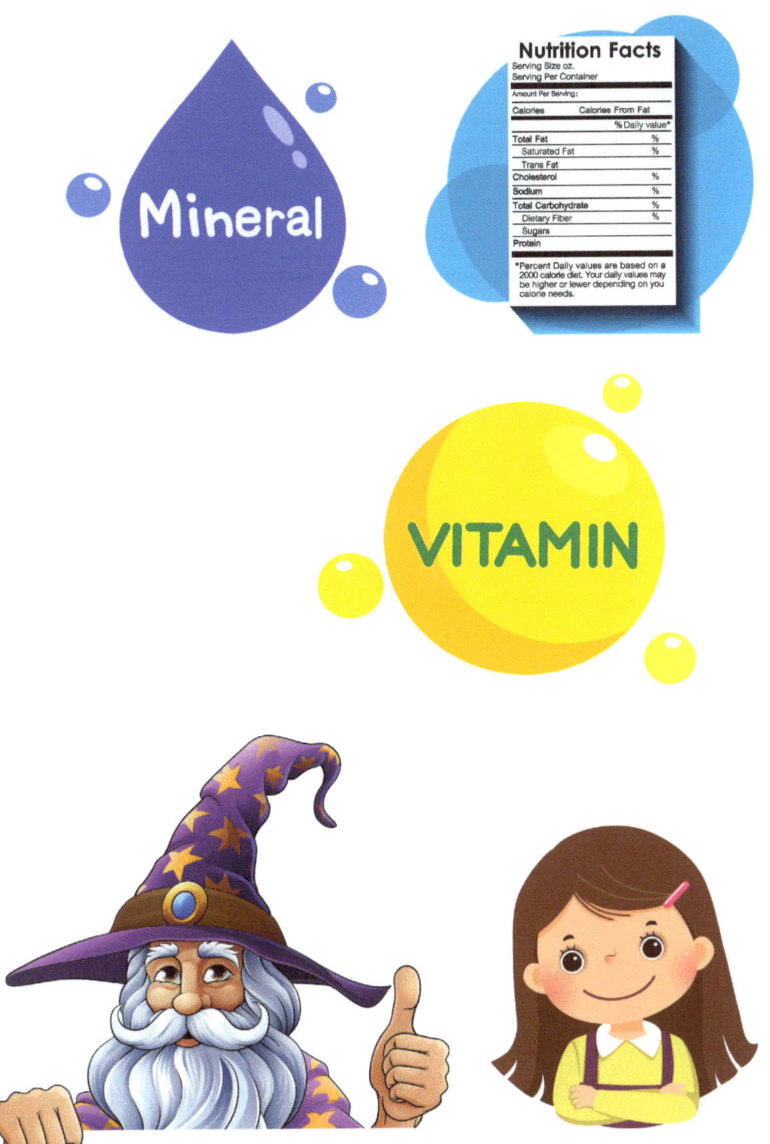

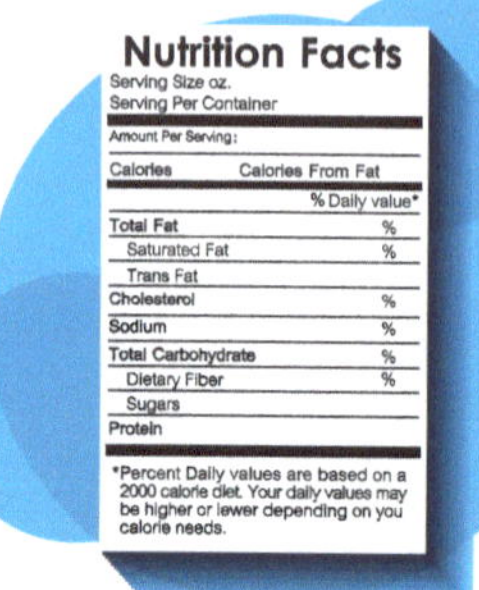

Macronutrients :
- Protein
- Fat
- Carbohydrates

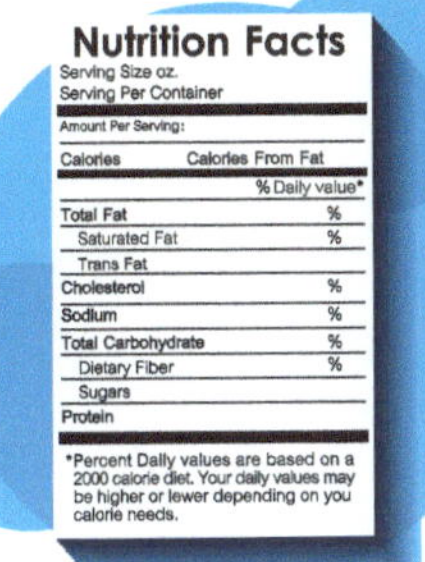

Micronutrients :
- **Minerals**
- **Vitamins**

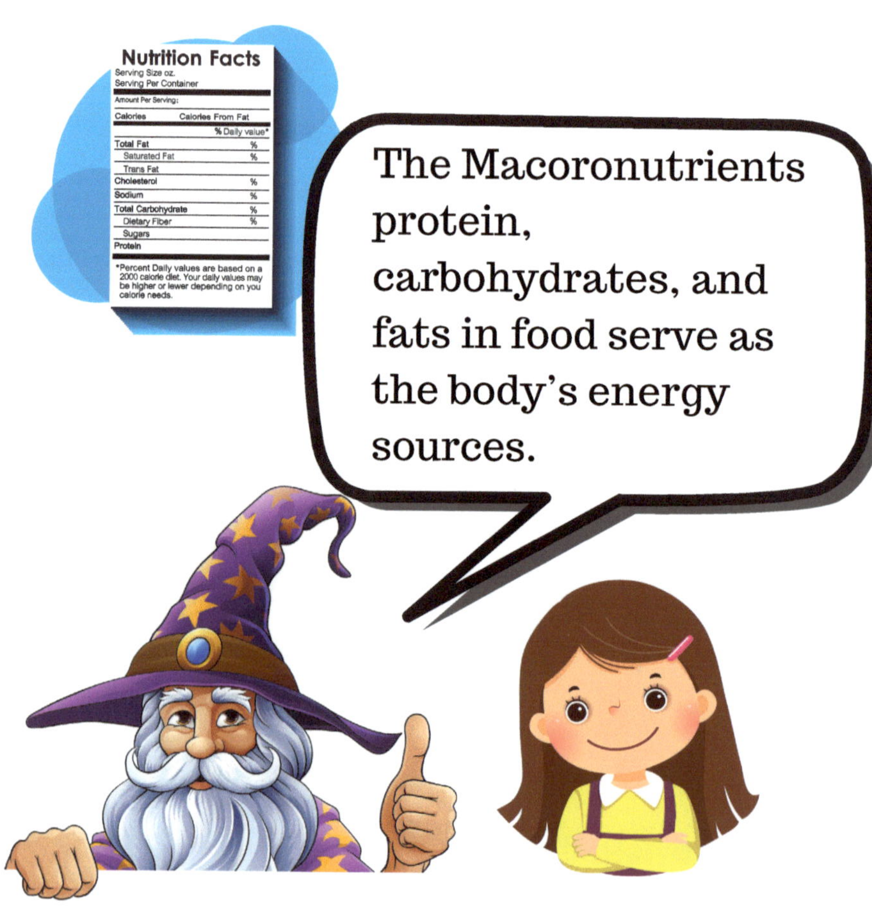

- Each gram of protein and carbohydrate supplies 4 calories, or units of energy.

- Fat contributes more than twice as much 9 calories per gram.

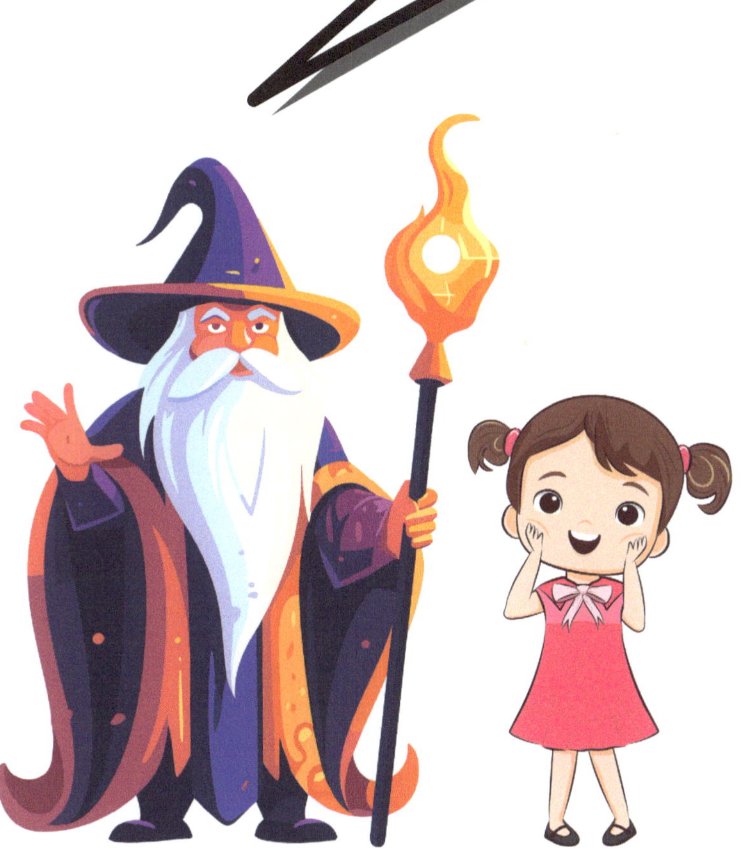

Calories are the measurement used to express the energy delivered by food.

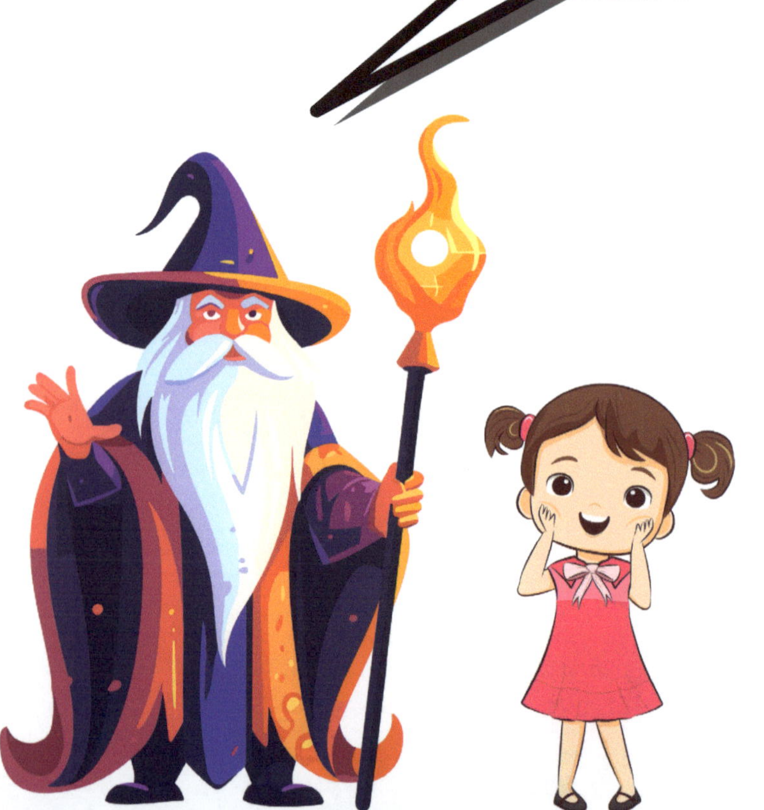

The body demands more calories during early adolescence than at any other time of life.

PROTEINS

YOGURT
Sources of protein are:
Beef, Chicken, Turkey,
Legumes, cheese, Milk,
Tofu, Yogurt, Fish,
Eggs

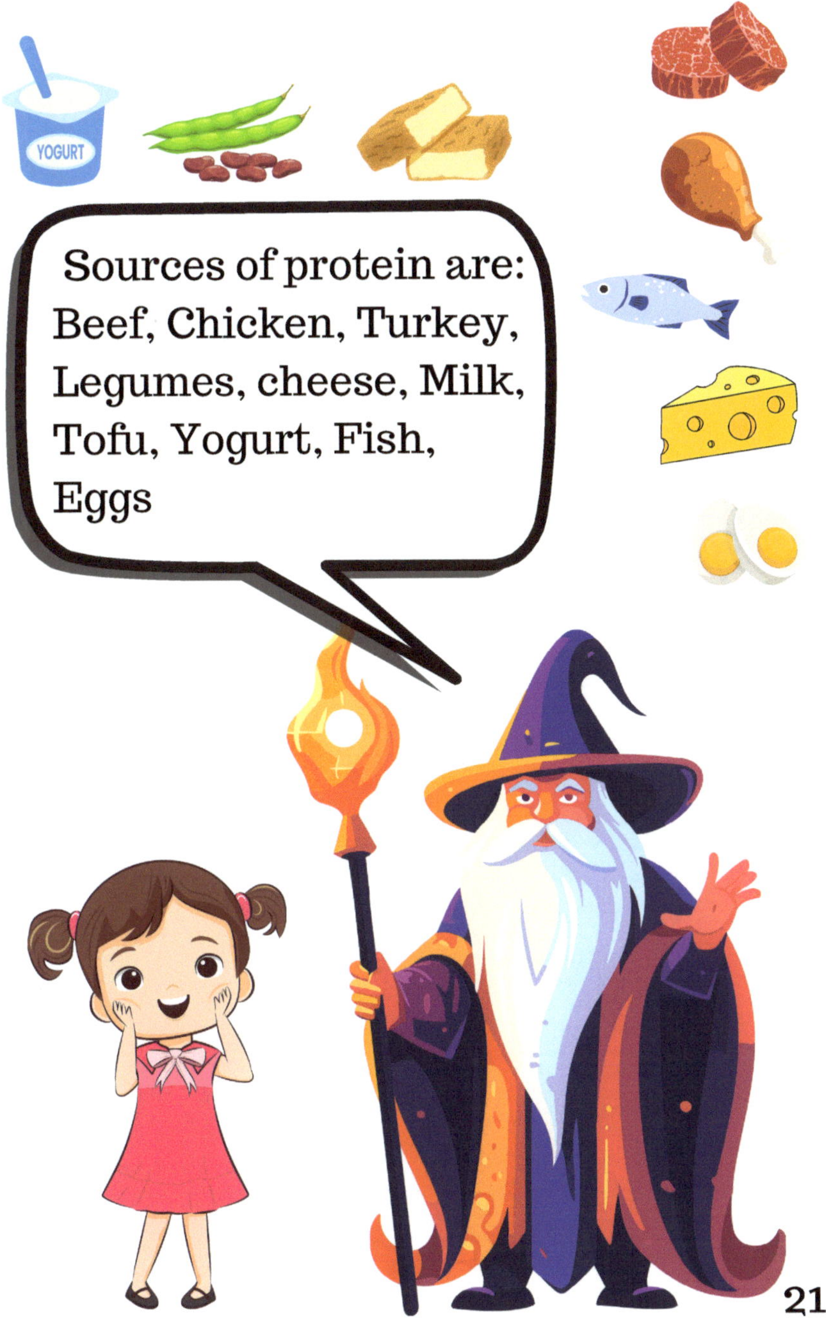

CARBOHYDRATES

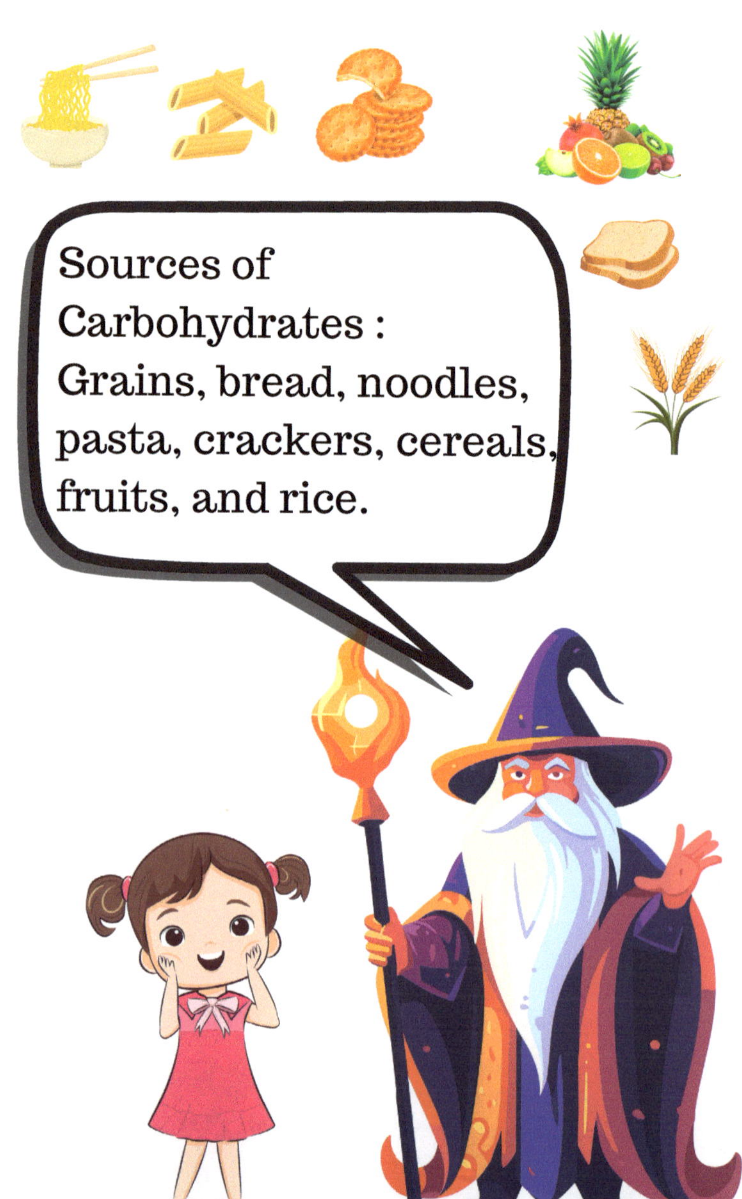

FATS

BUTTER

Sources of Fats:
Fatty fish, Eggs,
Avocado, Flaxseed,
Nuts and seed butter.

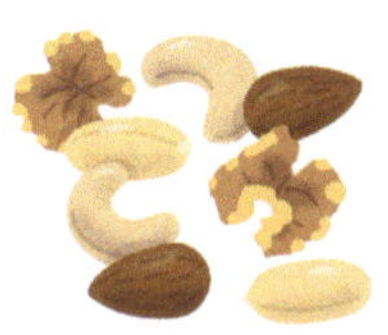

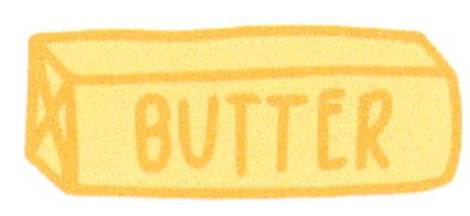

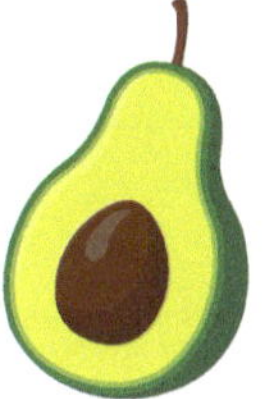

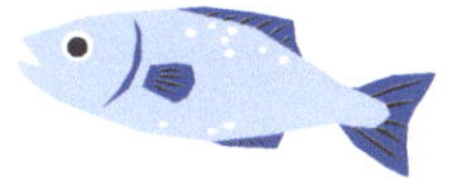

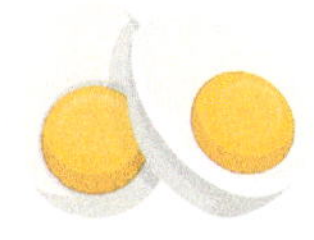

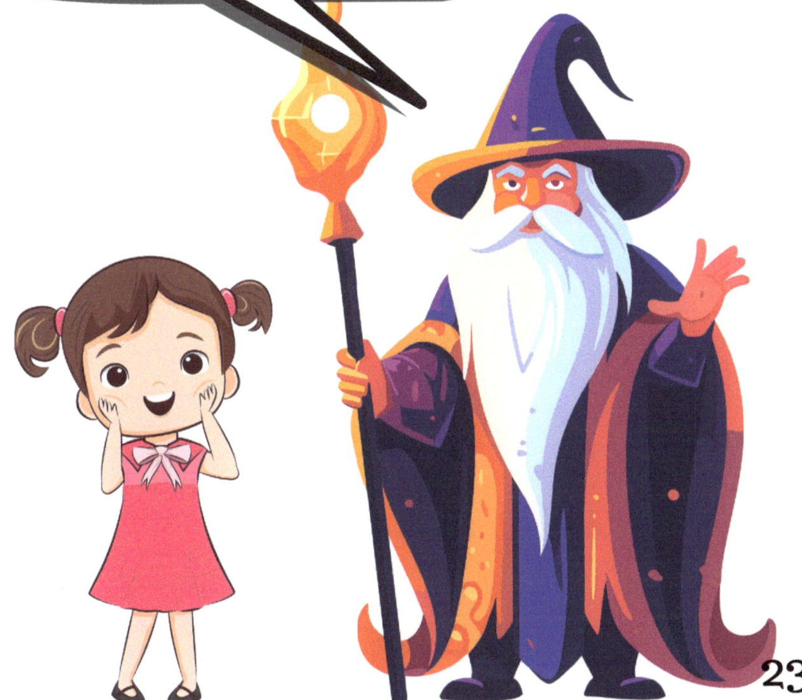

Ruhaani learned sources of food and useful tricks for identifying important numbers like serving sizes and percentages to help her choose healthier foods.

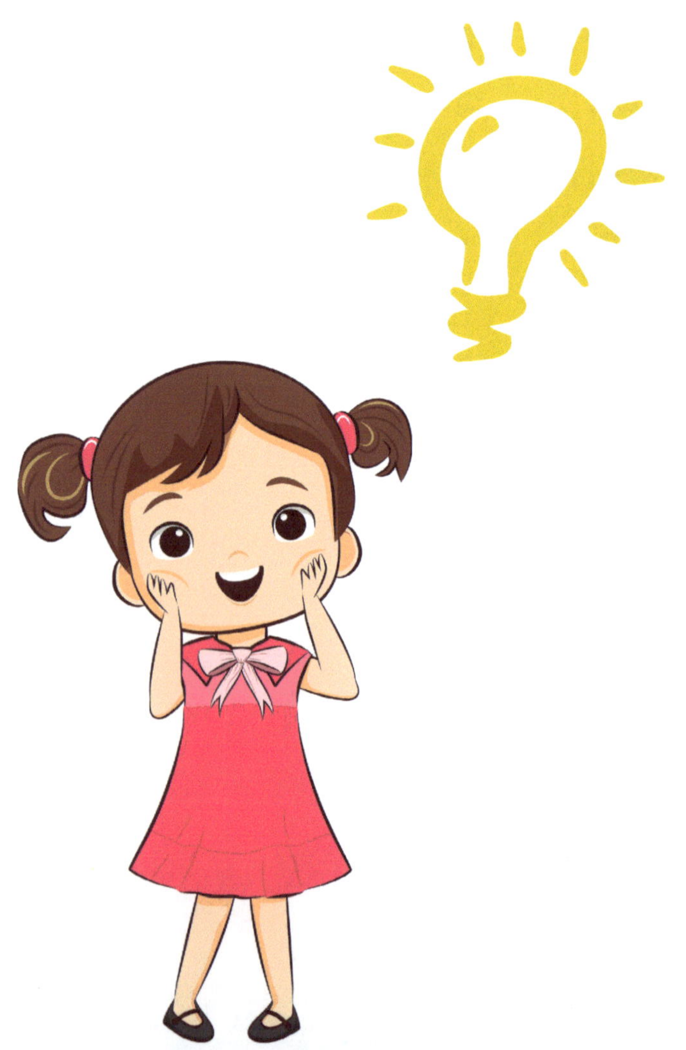

But there was one more mystery to solve - the Ingredients List.

The Ingredients List.

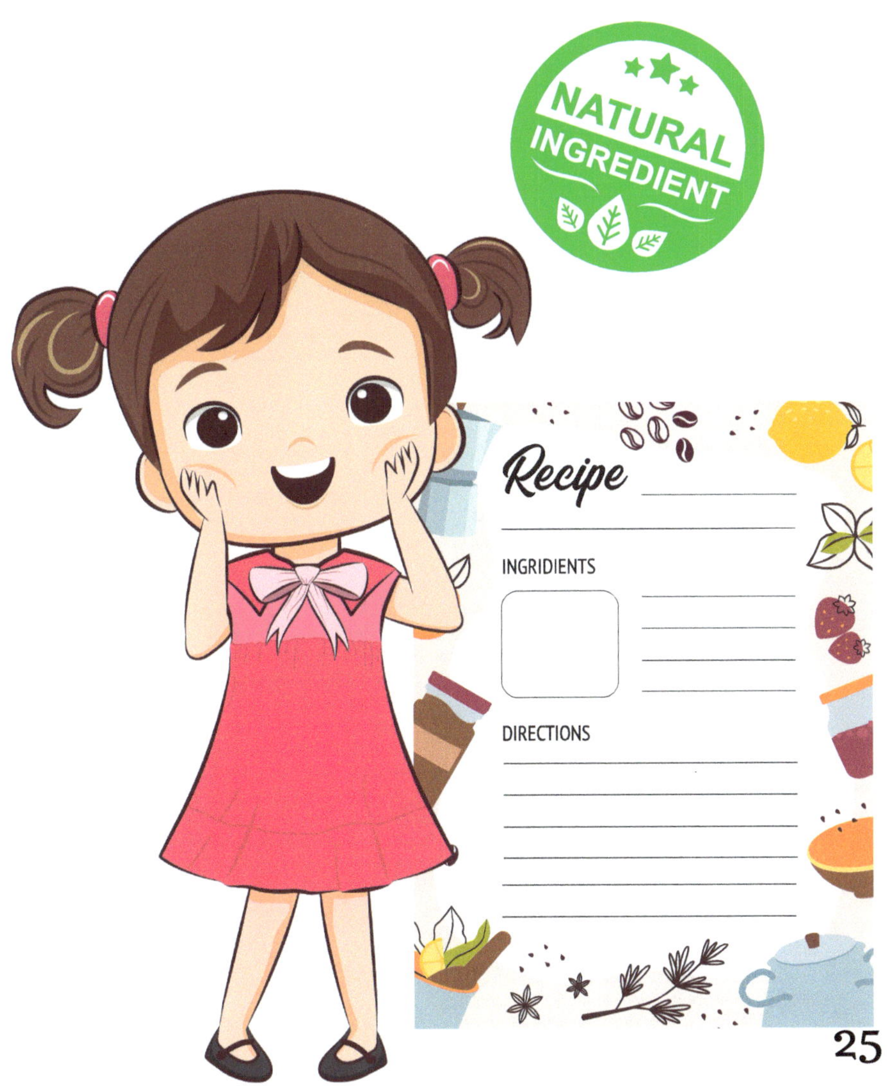

Rooh learned from the Nutrition Wizard how to read food labels to find out what ingredients were used.

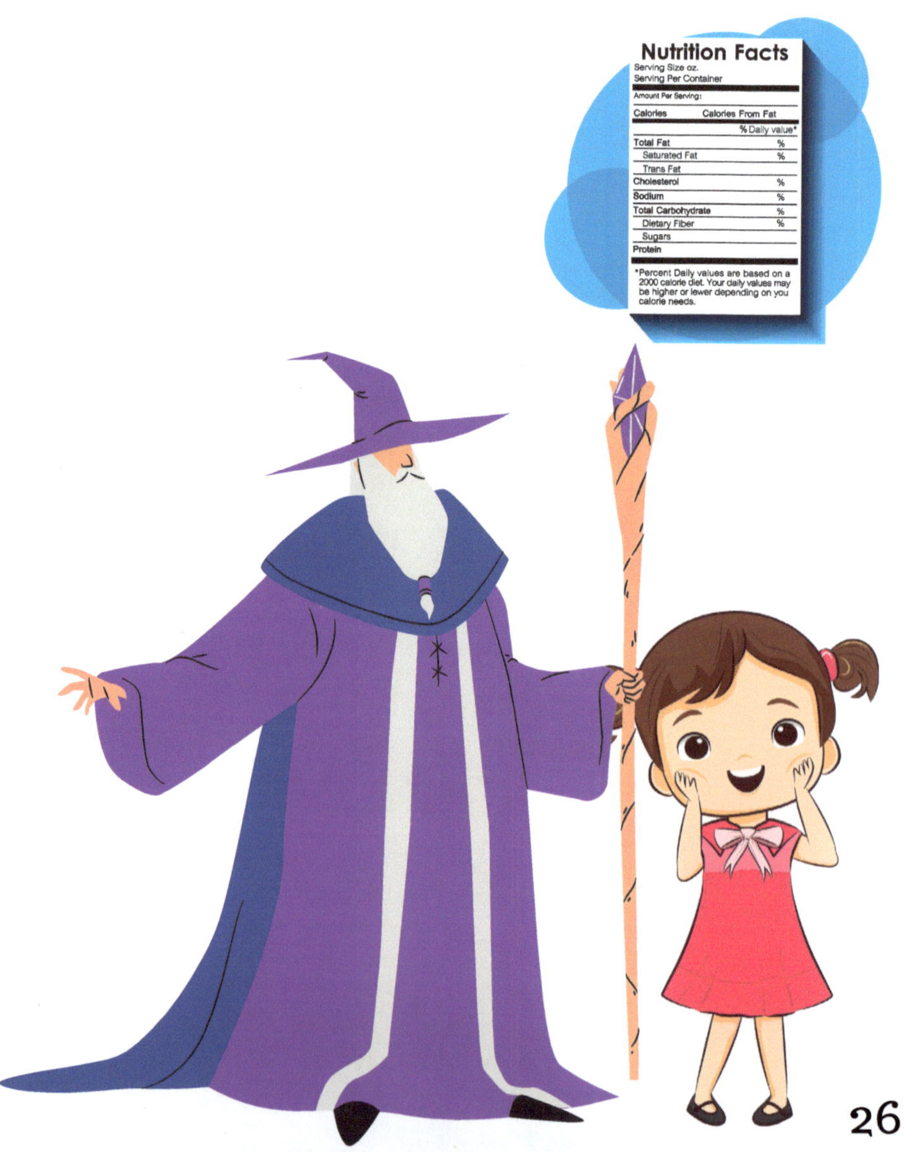

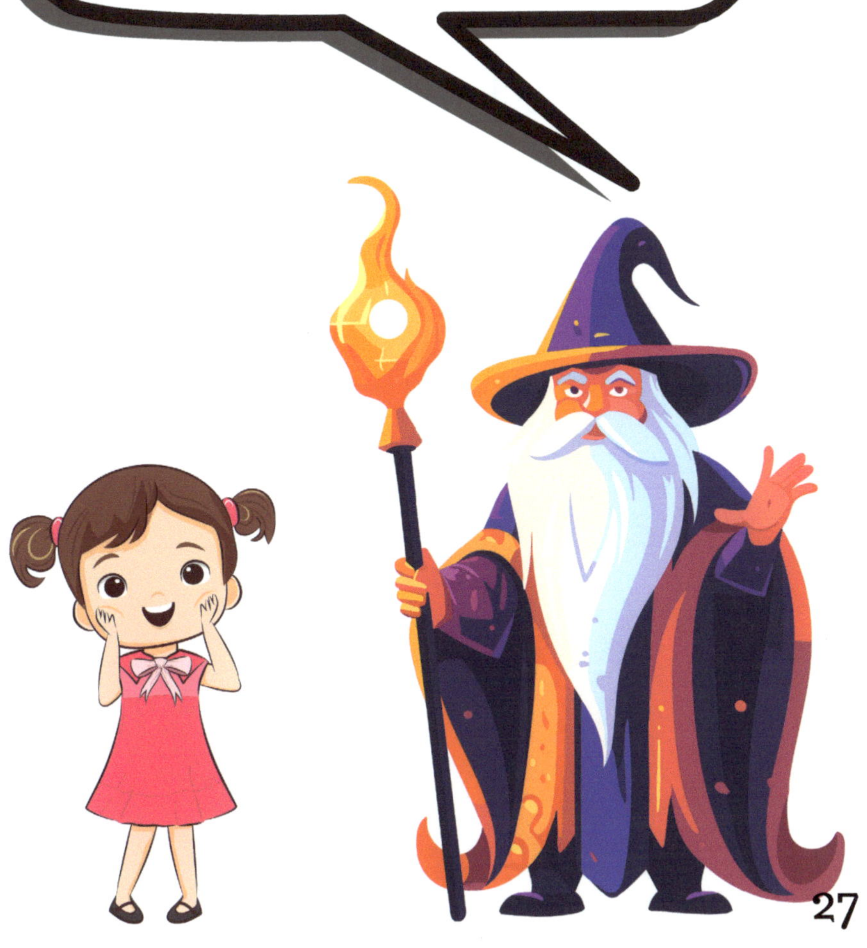
by simply looking at the length of an ingredient list, you can determine how processed a food is. Noting the number of additives it contains can give you a sense of the nutritional value even before you read the details.

Ingredients are listed in descending order by weight.
Focus on what comes first, but look further down the list, too.

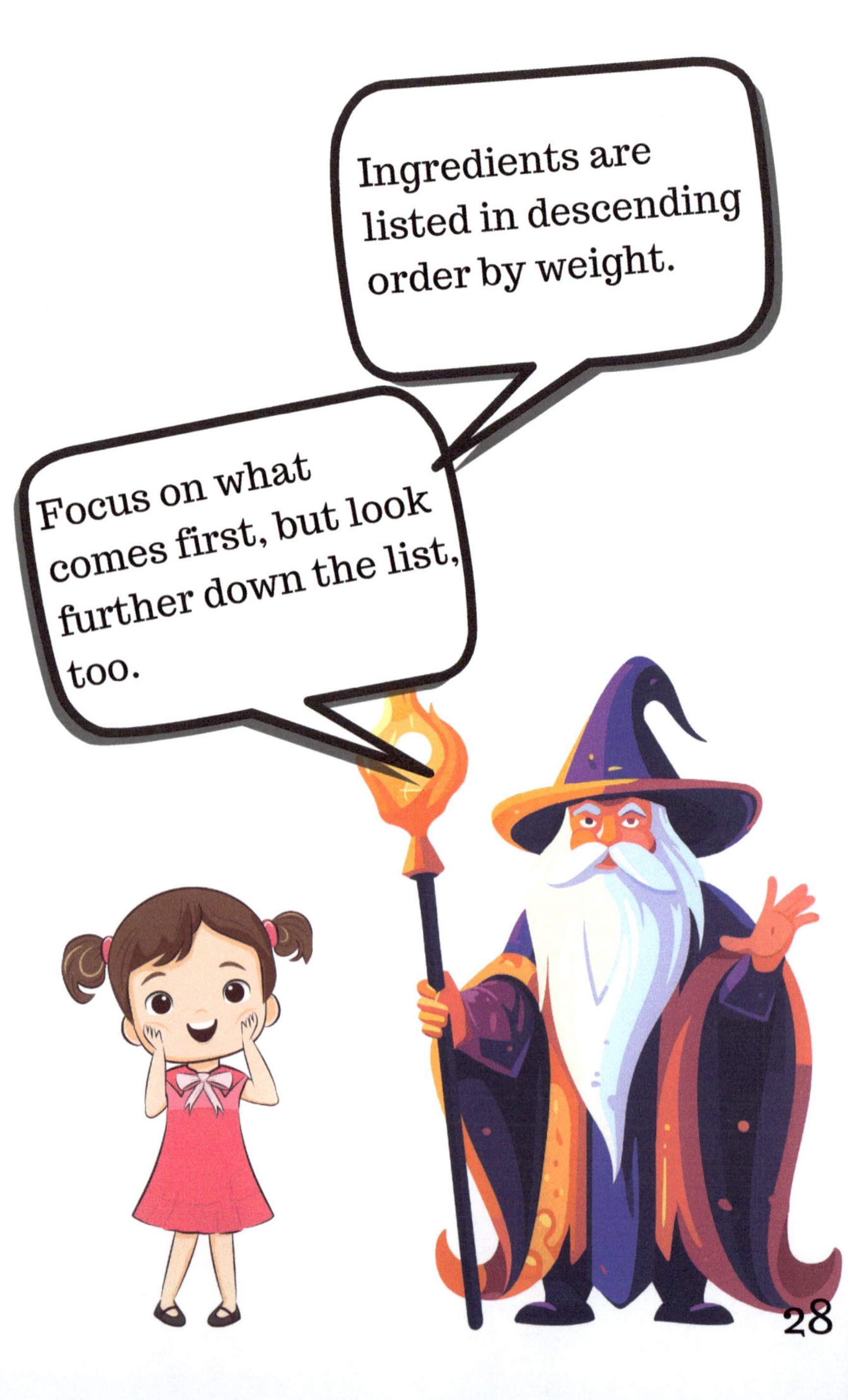

28

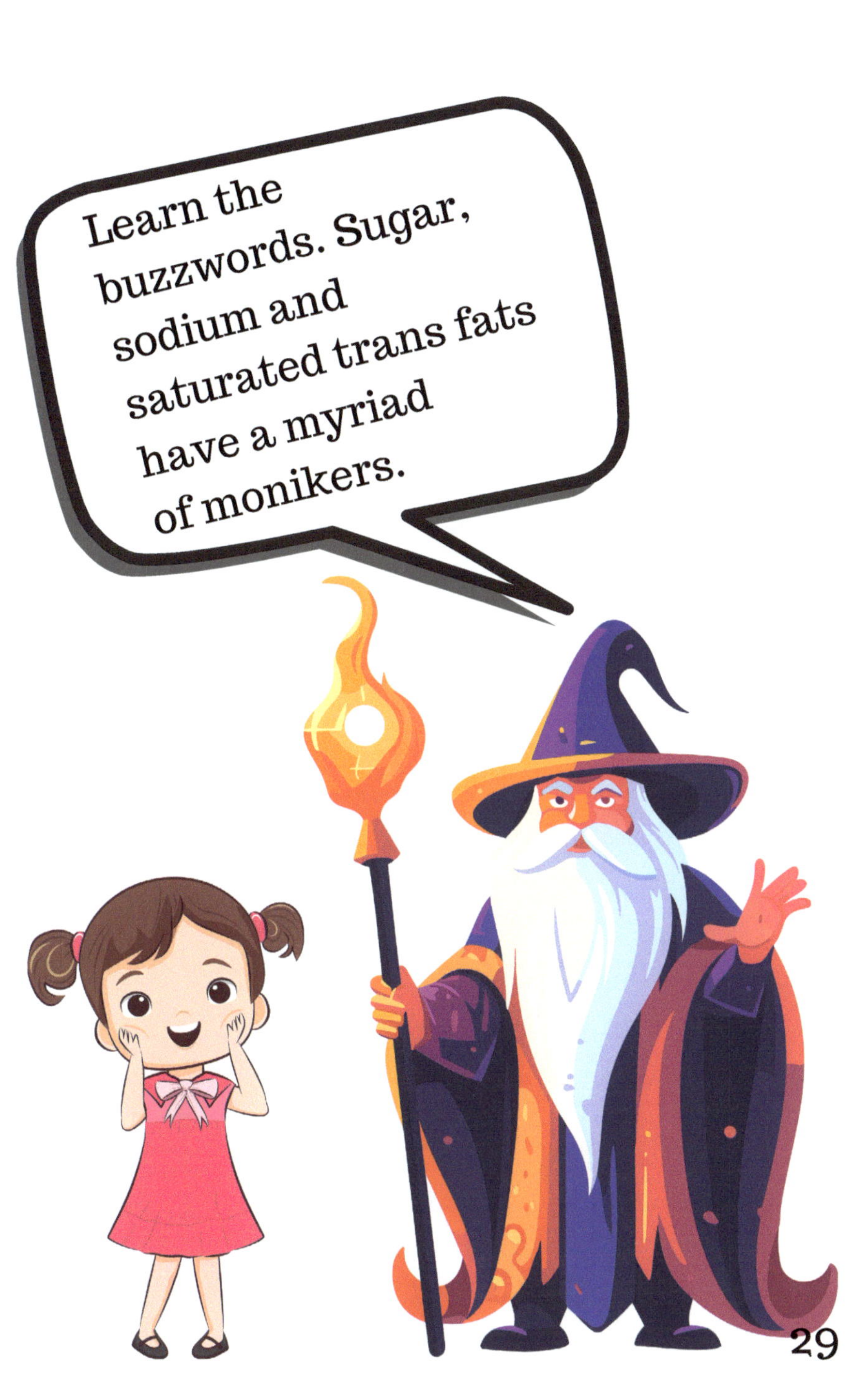

Learn the
buzzwords. Sugar,
sodium and
saturated trans fats
have a myriad
of monikers.

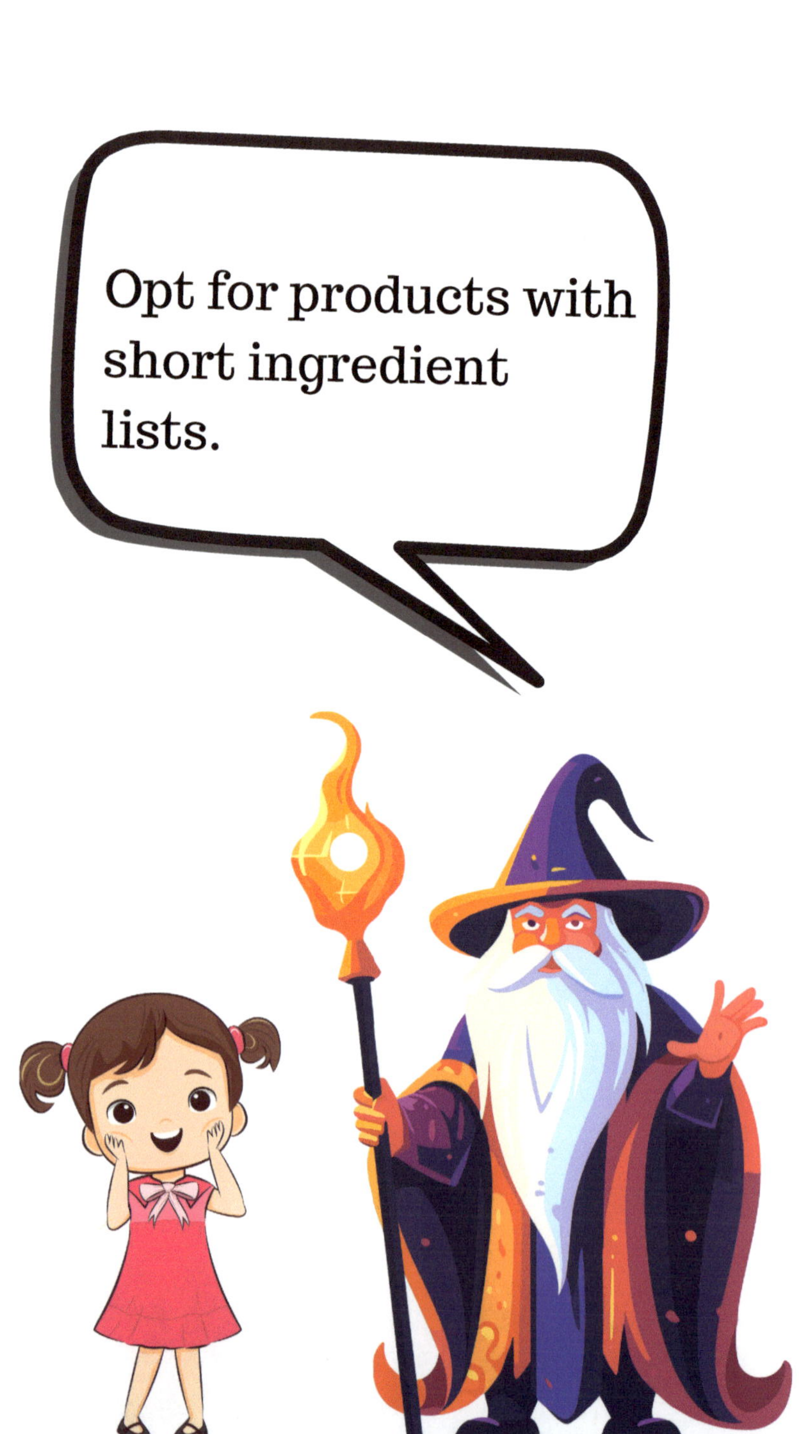
Opt for products with short ingredient lists.

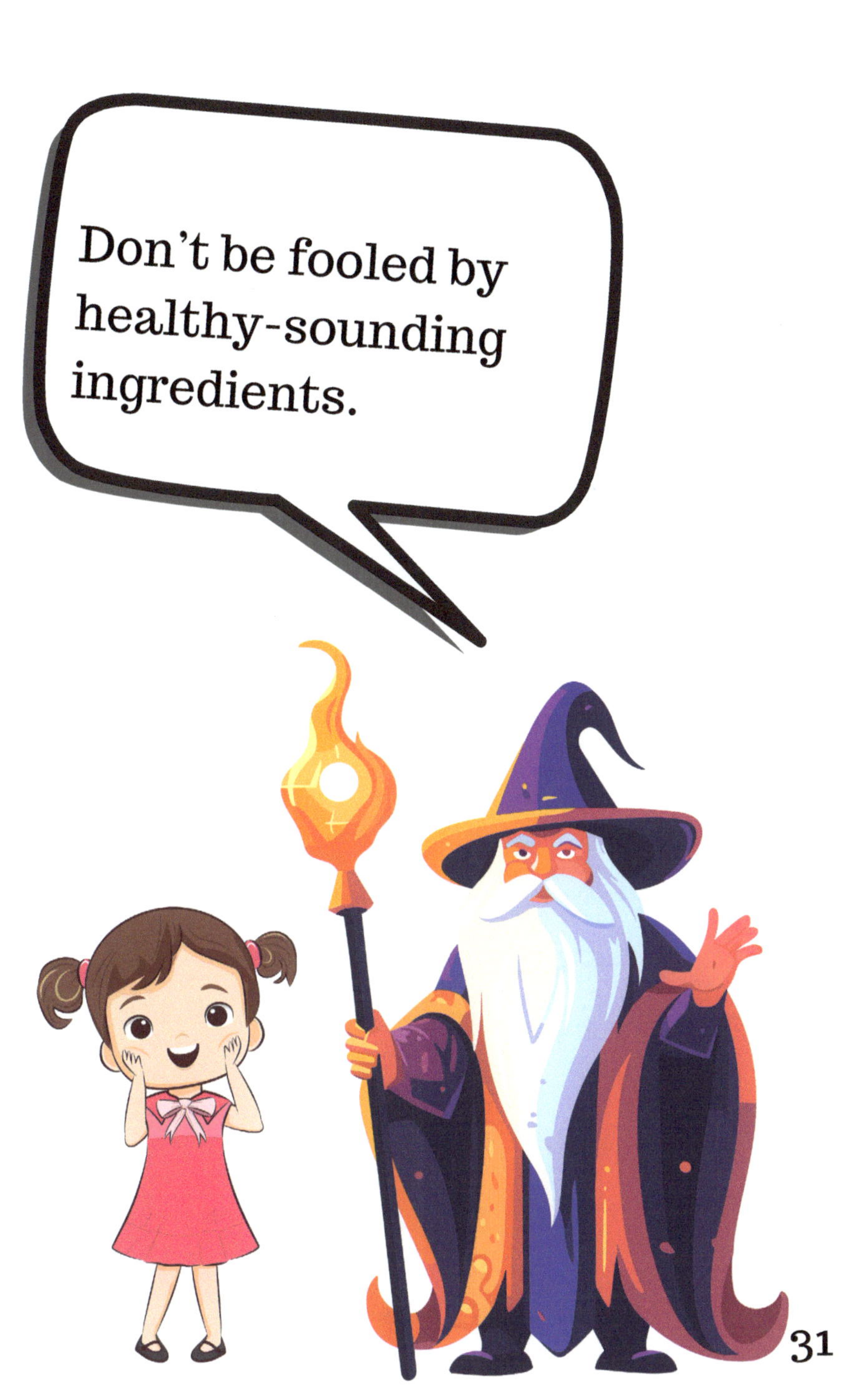

Don't be fooled by healthy-sounding ingredients.

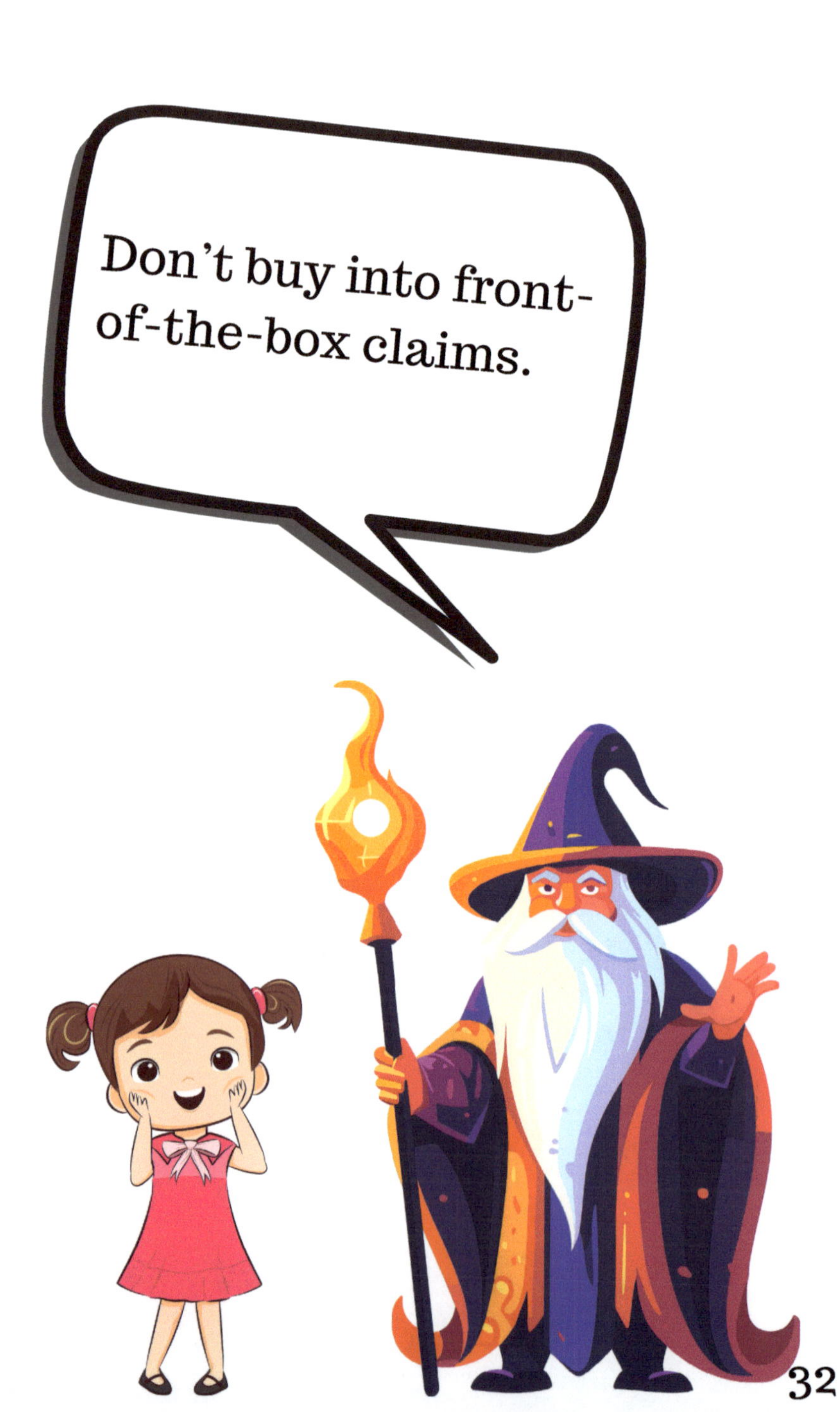
Don't buy into front-of-the-box claims.

They realized that choosing foods with simple, natural ingredients is best for staying healthy, and to avoid those with long and complicated names. Avoid foods with artificial colors and preservatives.

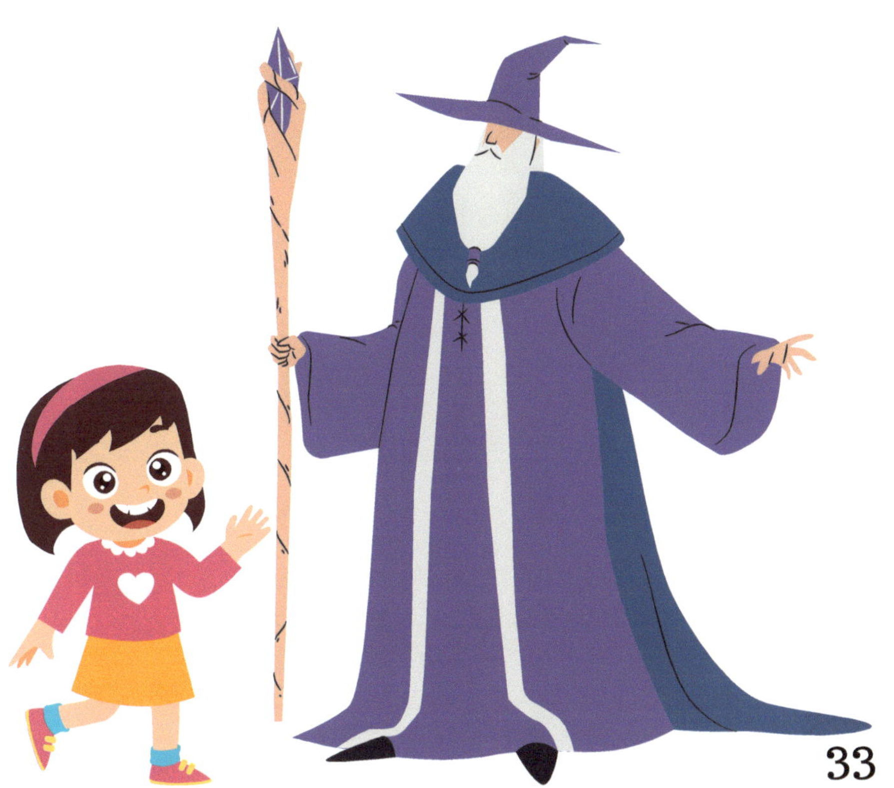

Ruhaani was excited to learn how to read nutrition labels and ingredients. She felt confident to make healthy choices for her well-being.

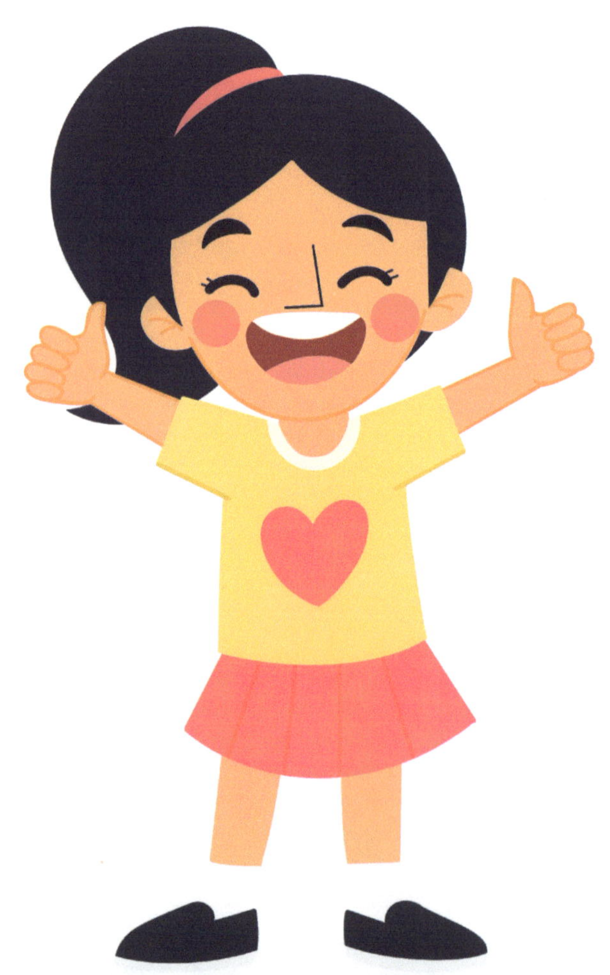

A wizard told her about gut health and
how 90% of our immune system resides
in gut.

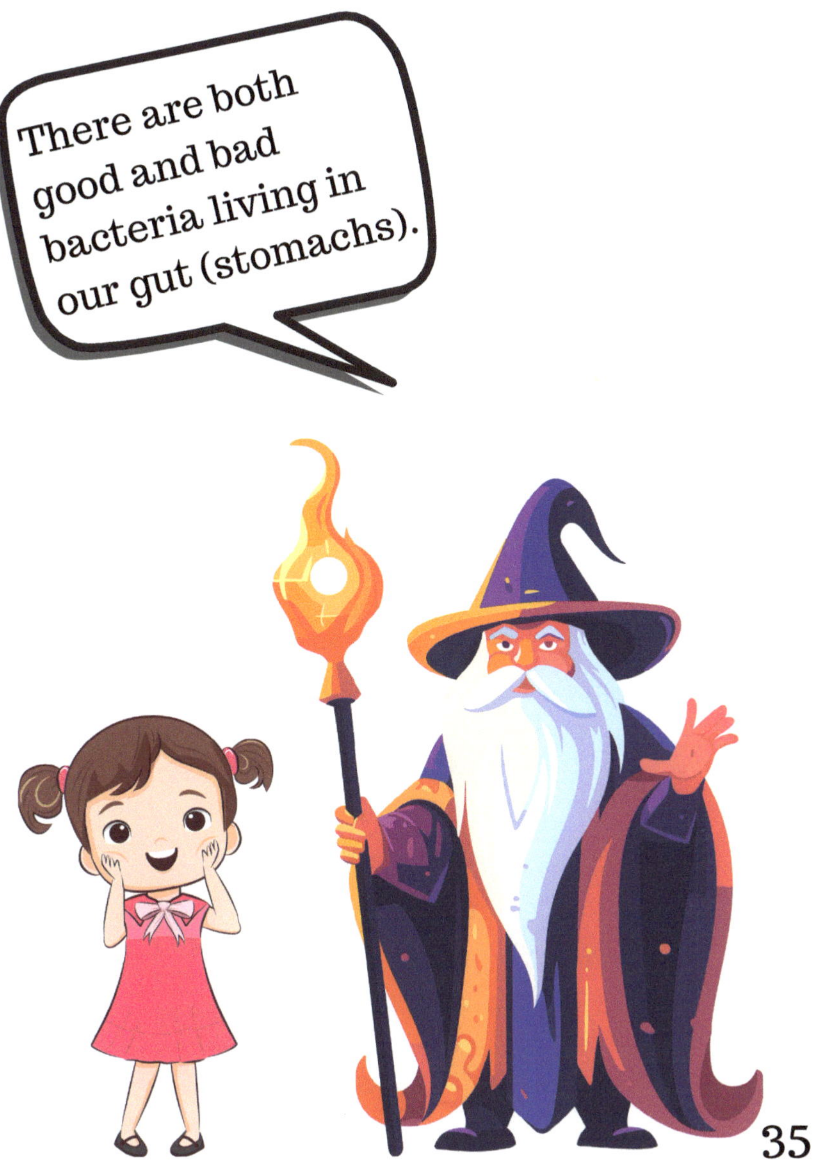

Good bacteria like Lactobacillus and Bifidobacterium help with digestion and boost our immune system.

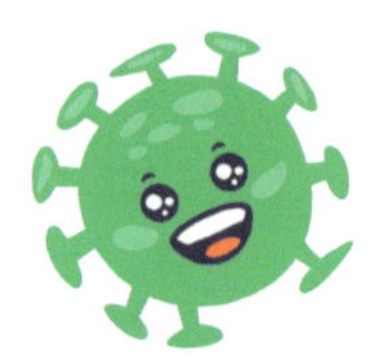

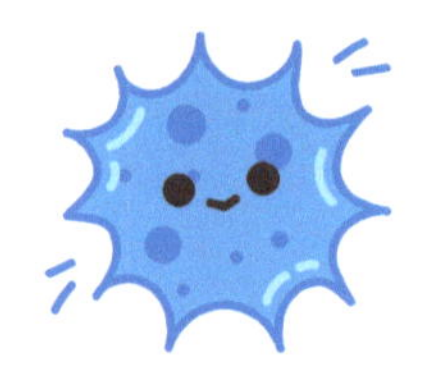

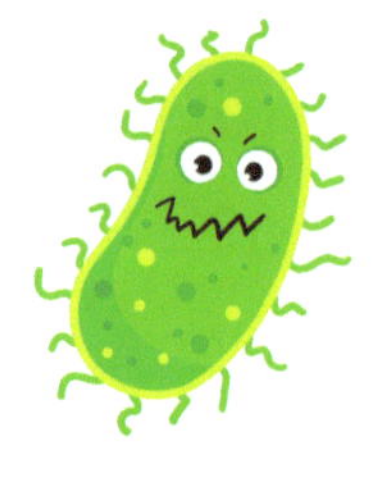

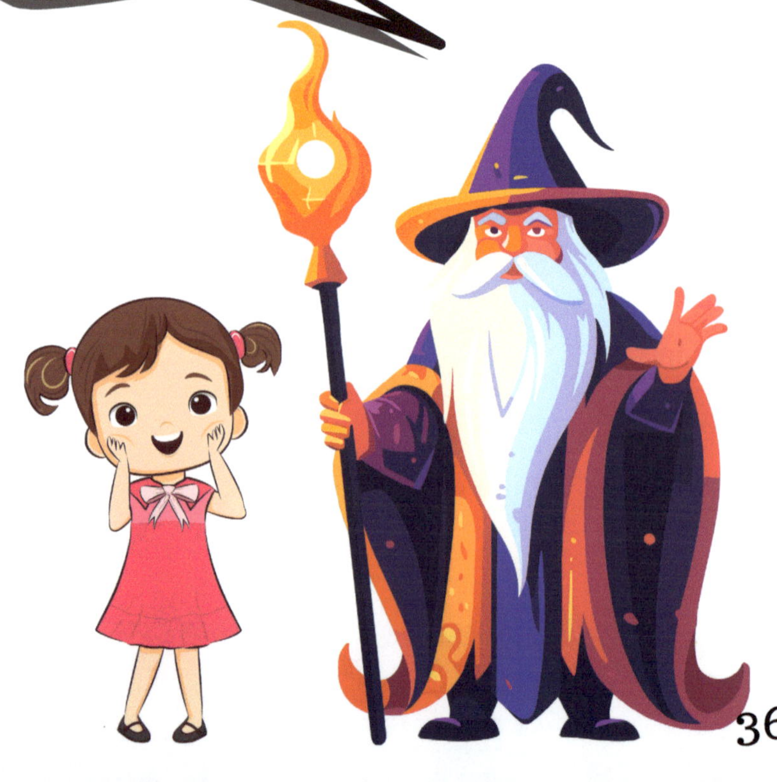

36

We can help these friendly
bacteria by eating foods like
yogurt, kefir,
Kombucha, and other fermented
foods (Probiotics)

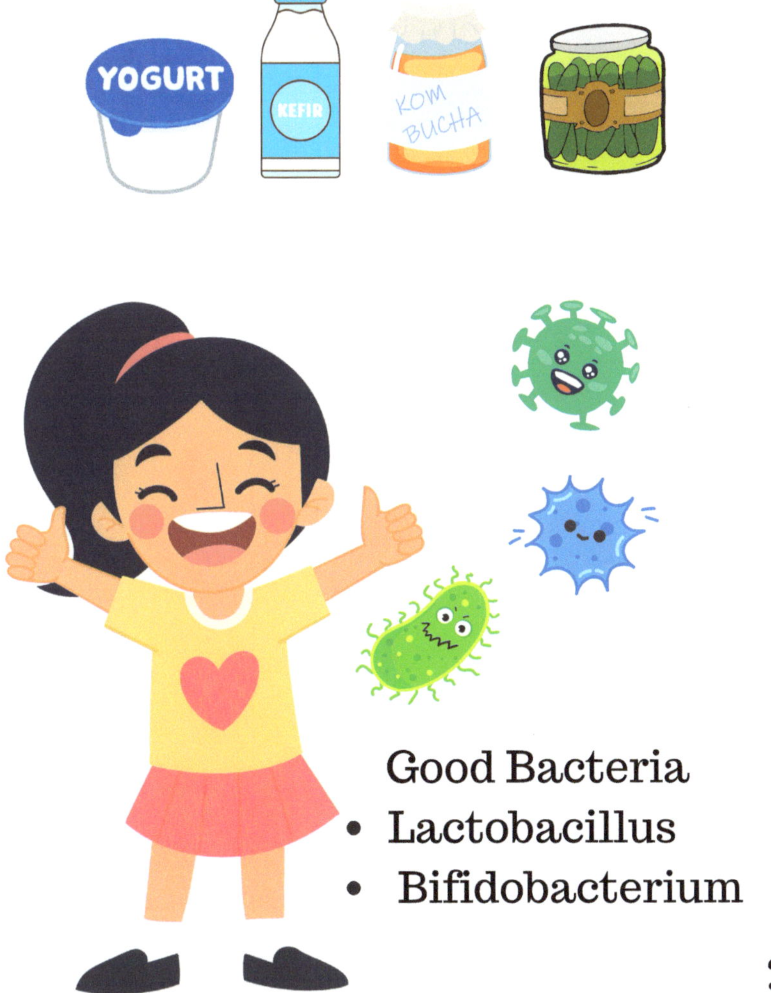

Good Bacteria
- Lactobacillus
- Bifidobacterium

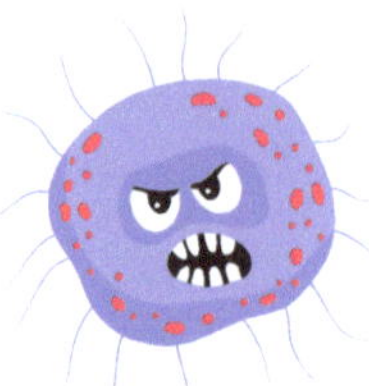
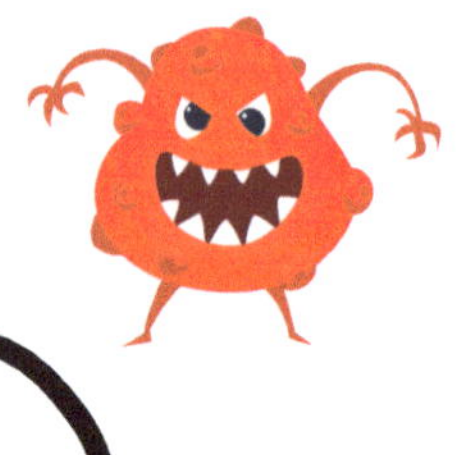
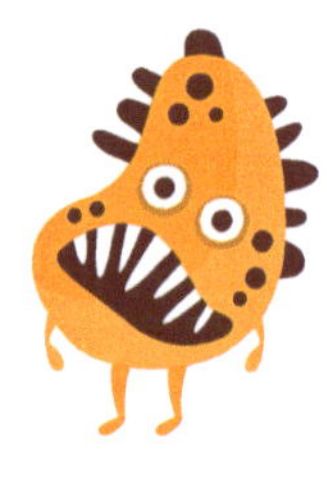
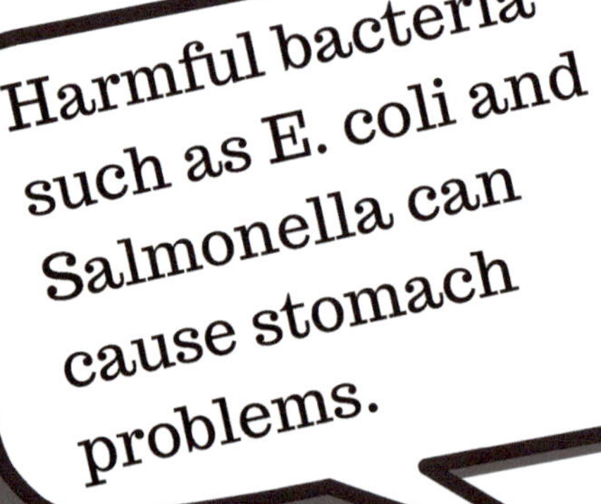

Harmful bacteria such as E. coli and Salmonella can cause stomach problems.

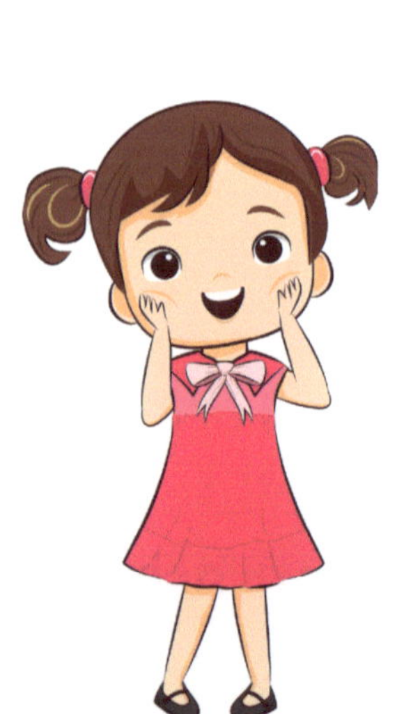
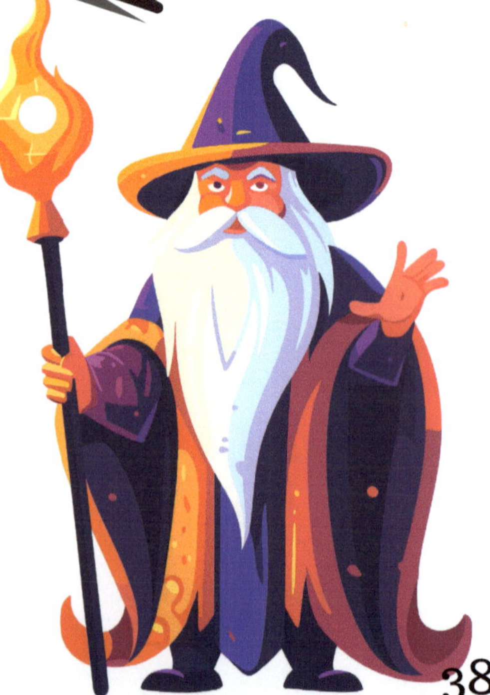

To prevent these bacteria, avoid eating sugary and processed foods they like.

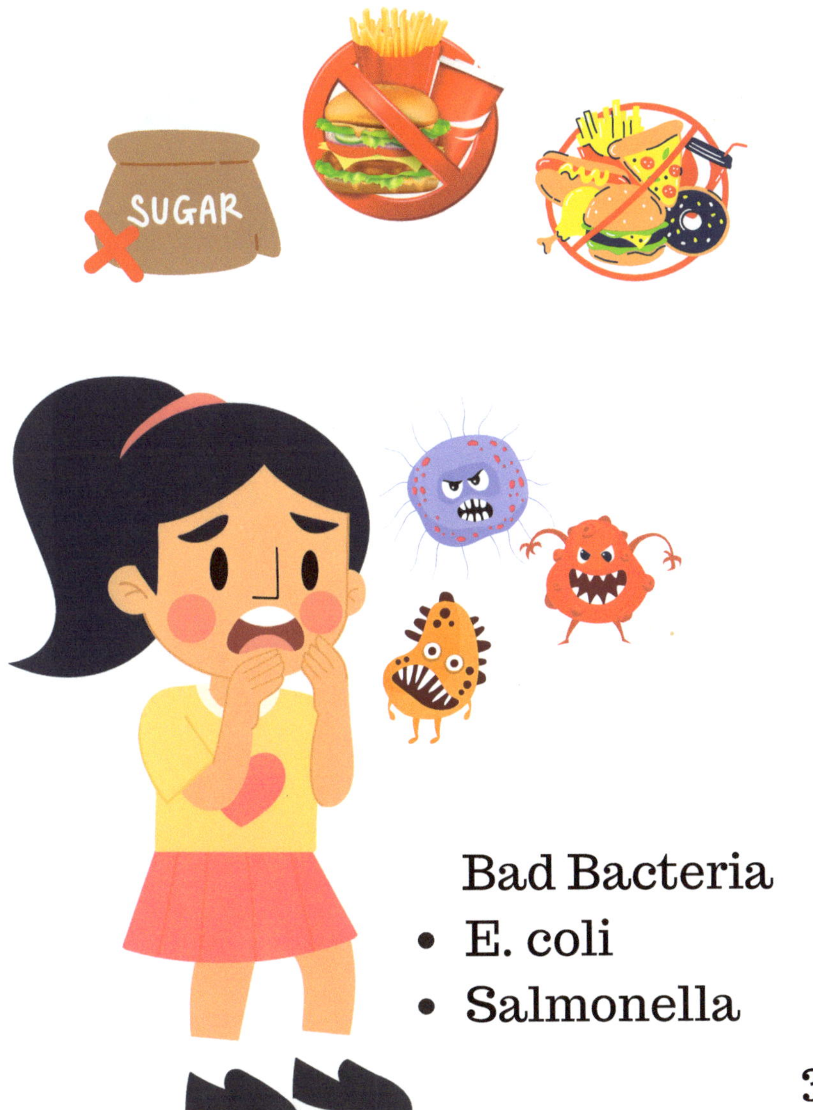

Rooh was pleased that she can now understand sugar labels, colors, artificial sweeteners.

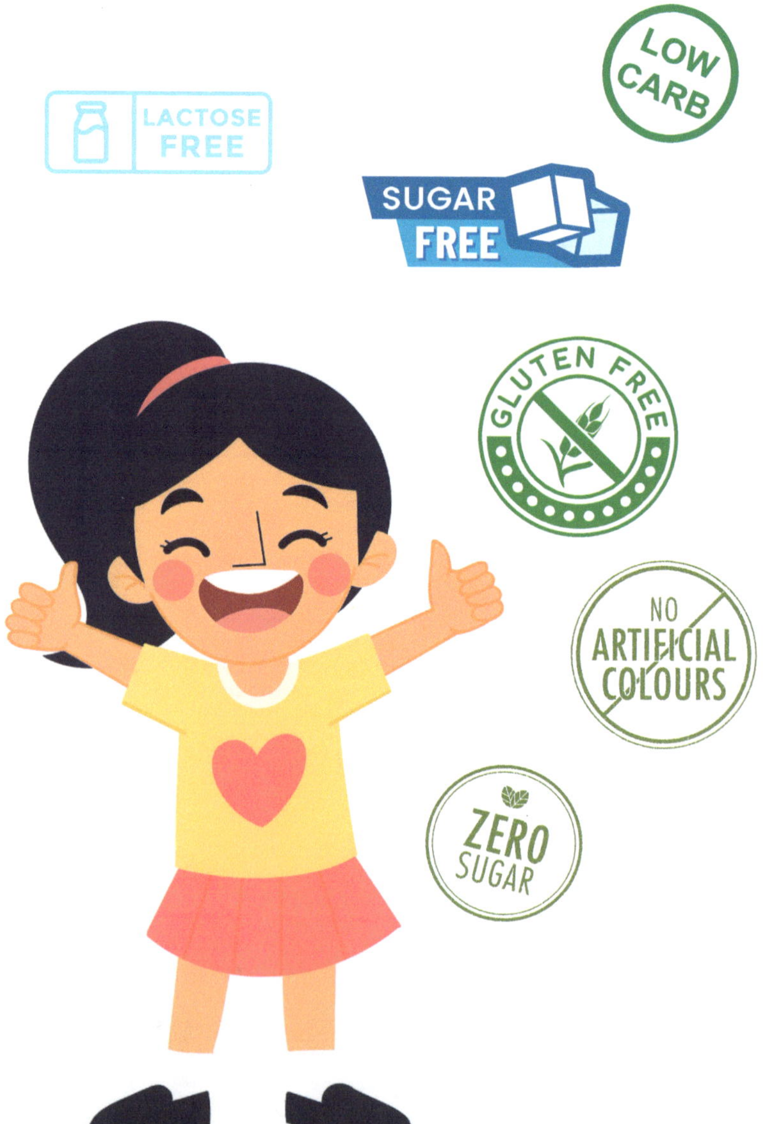

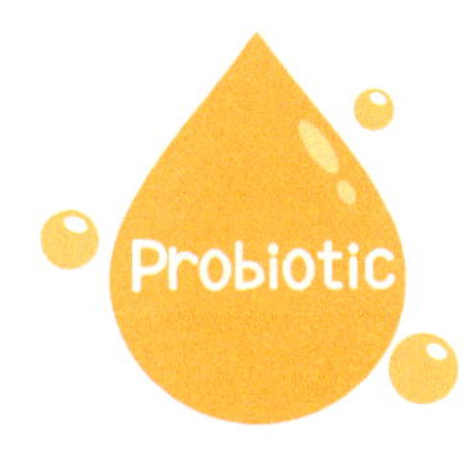

Probiotic

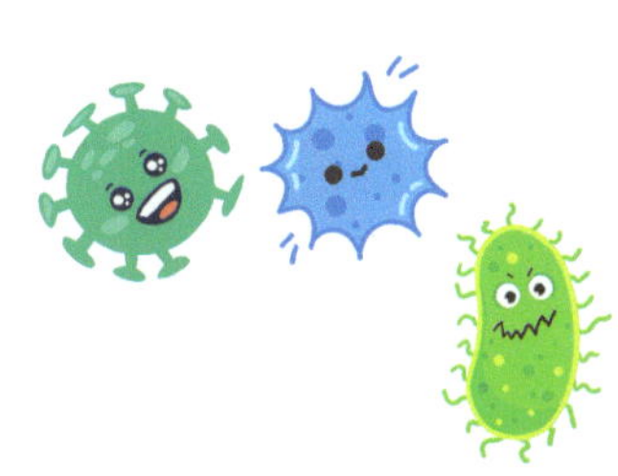

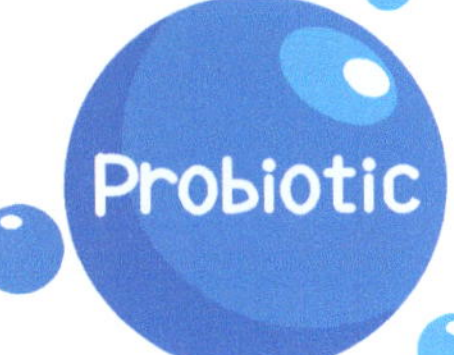

Probiotic

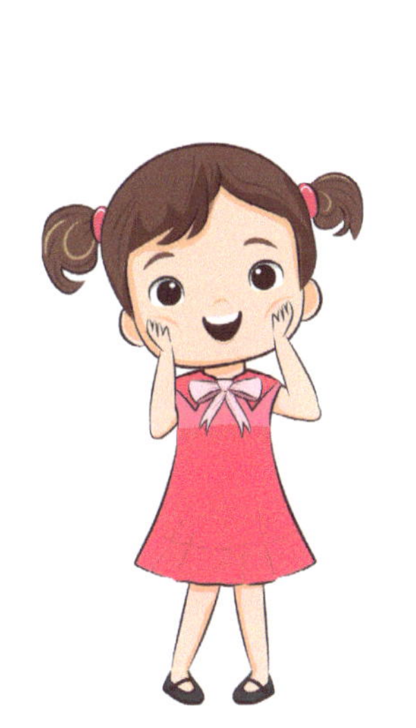

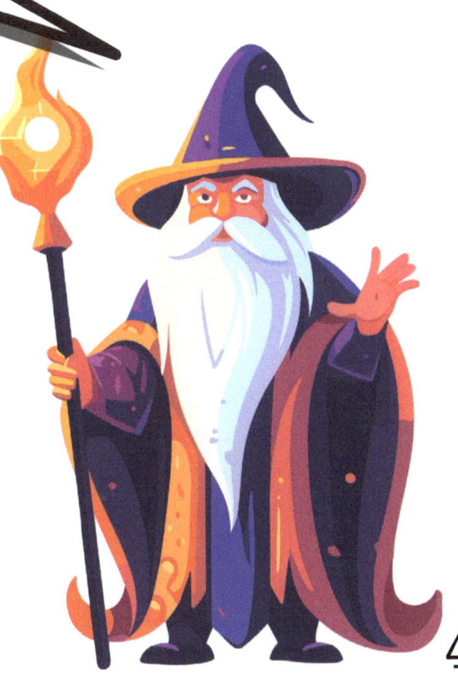

Don't forget to nourish your beneficial bacteria with healthy, fiber-rich foods also called prebiotics,

Drink lots of water, and stay active to keep your gut healthy and your body in good shape!

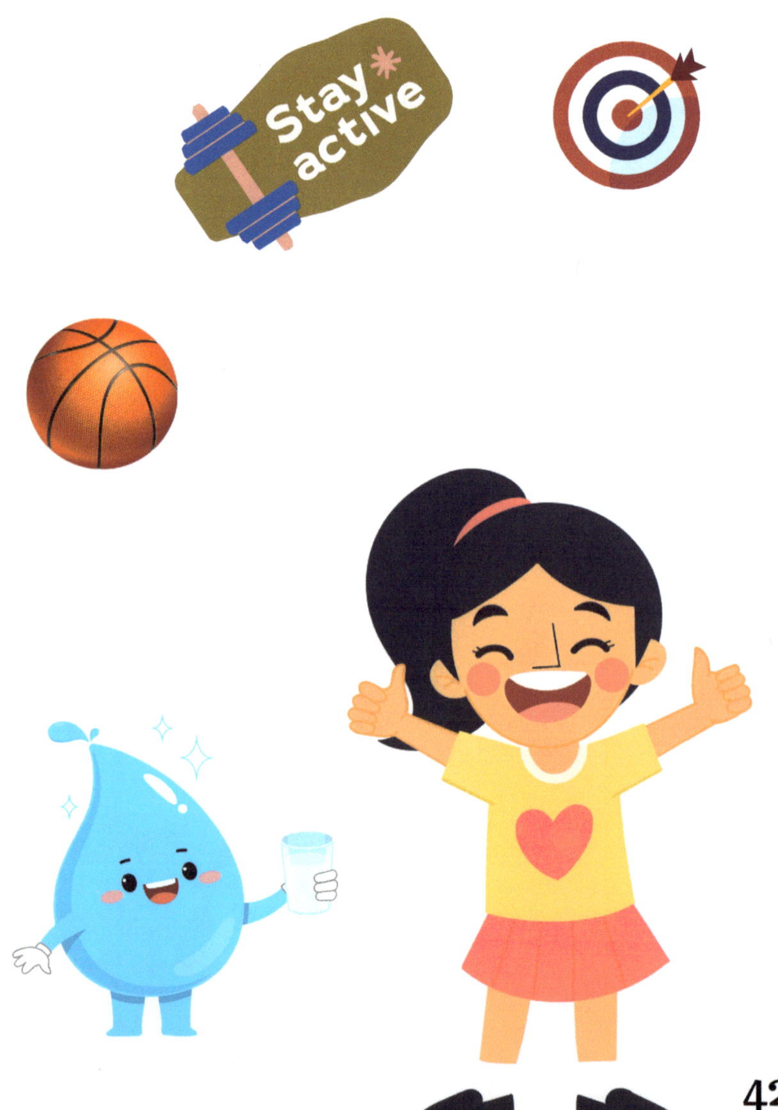

Starting from that day, Ruhaani was called the Nutrition Queen of Nutraville.

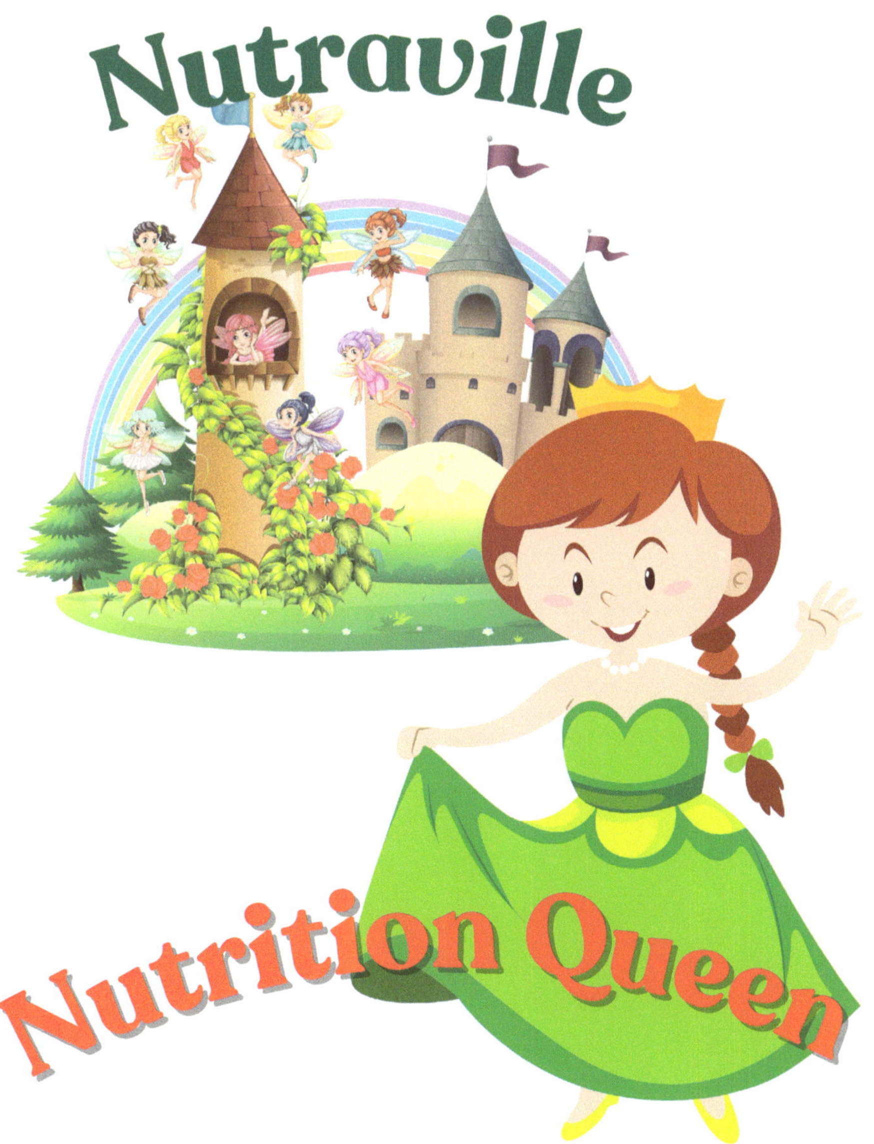

She shared her knowledge with those who wanted to eat healthily.

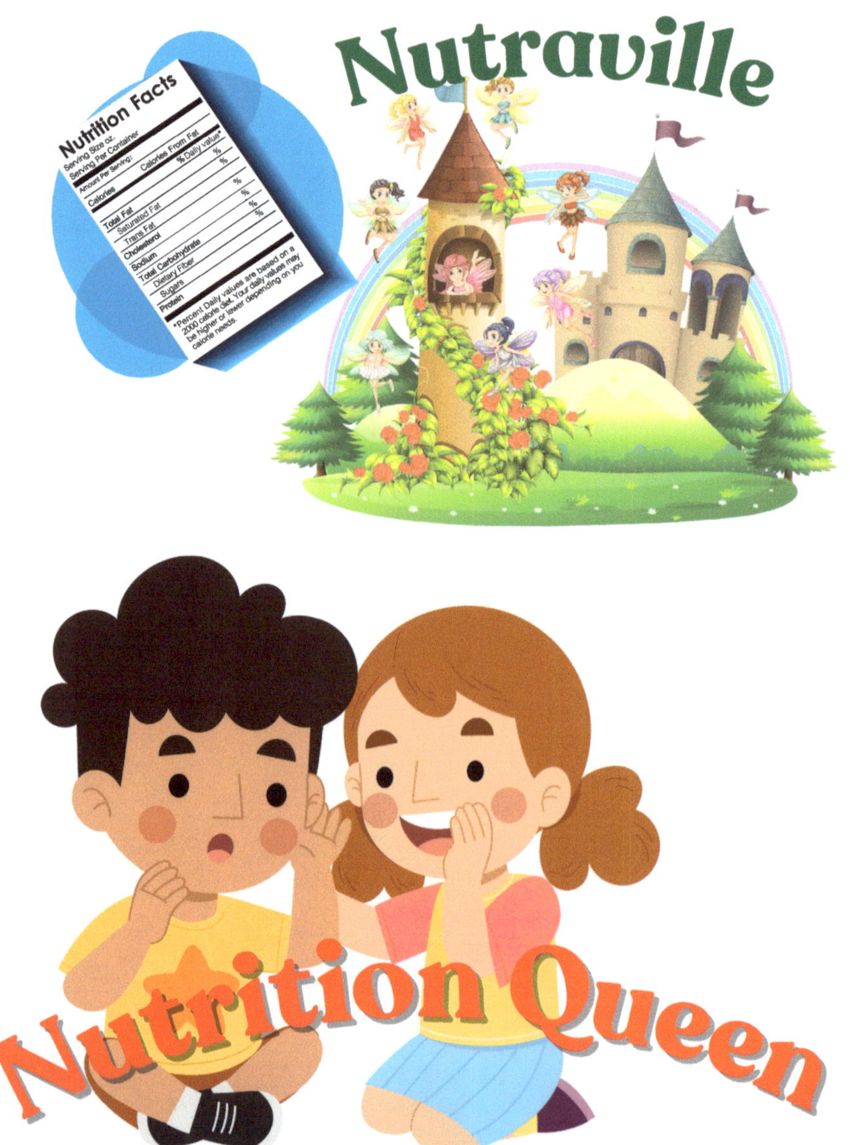

44

Ruhaani discovered that by reading nutrition labels and ingredients, she could understand the secrets of the foods she ate and lead a healthy, happy life.

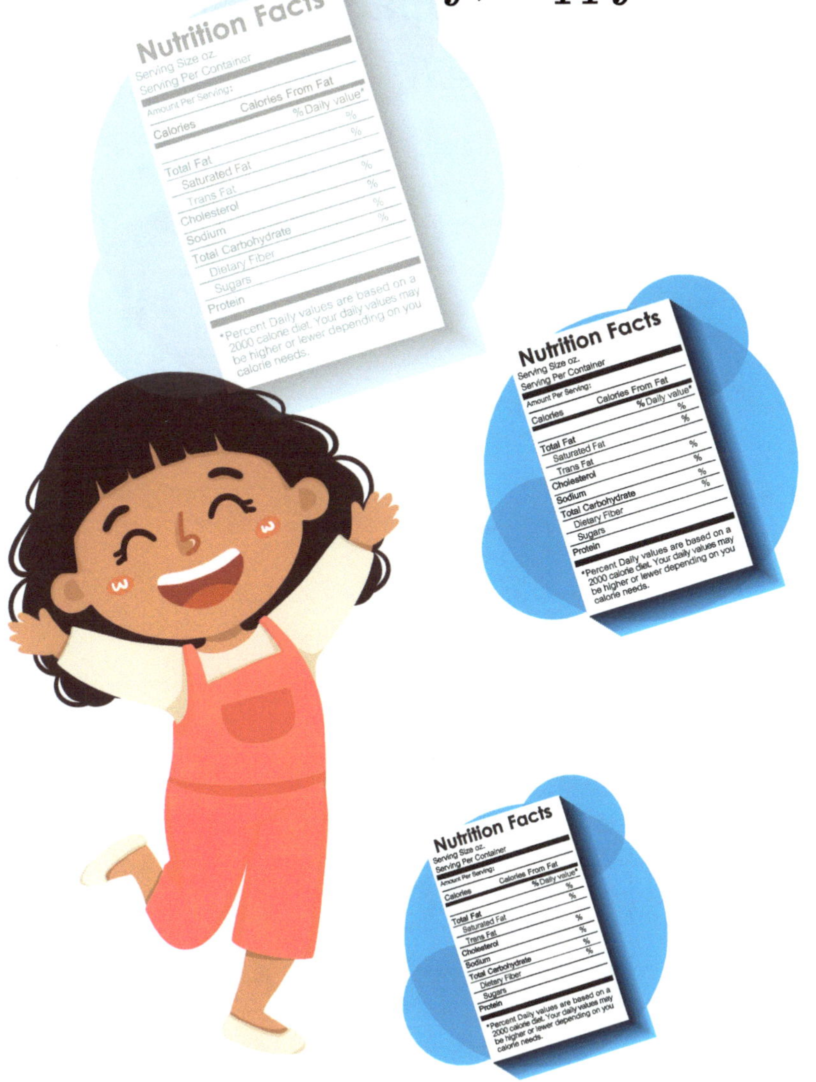

45

She learned to read nutrition labels accurately, understanding serving sizes and ingredients clearly. Colors and numbers that used to be confusing to her now made sense, showing her the impact of the food she ate on her body.

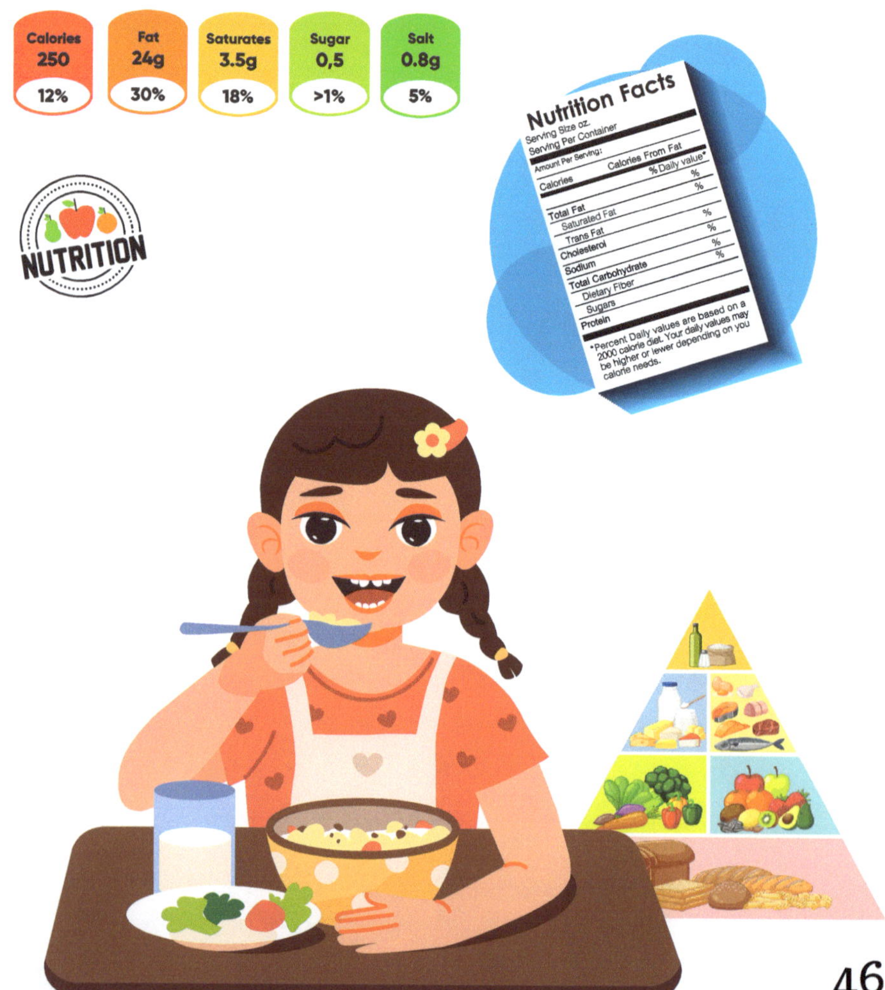

With this new knowledge and a strong sense of purpose, Ruhaani took control of her nutrition like never before. She carefully examined every label, ingredient, and calorie to ensure that each bite she took helped her health and energy.

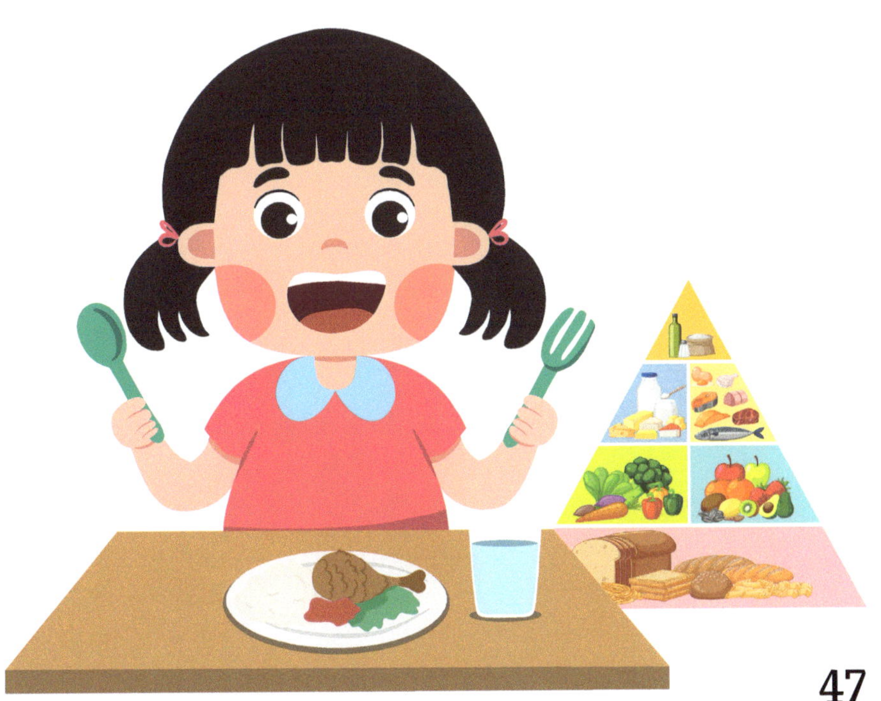

She monitored her food closely, focusing on the nutrients that supported her passions and goals.

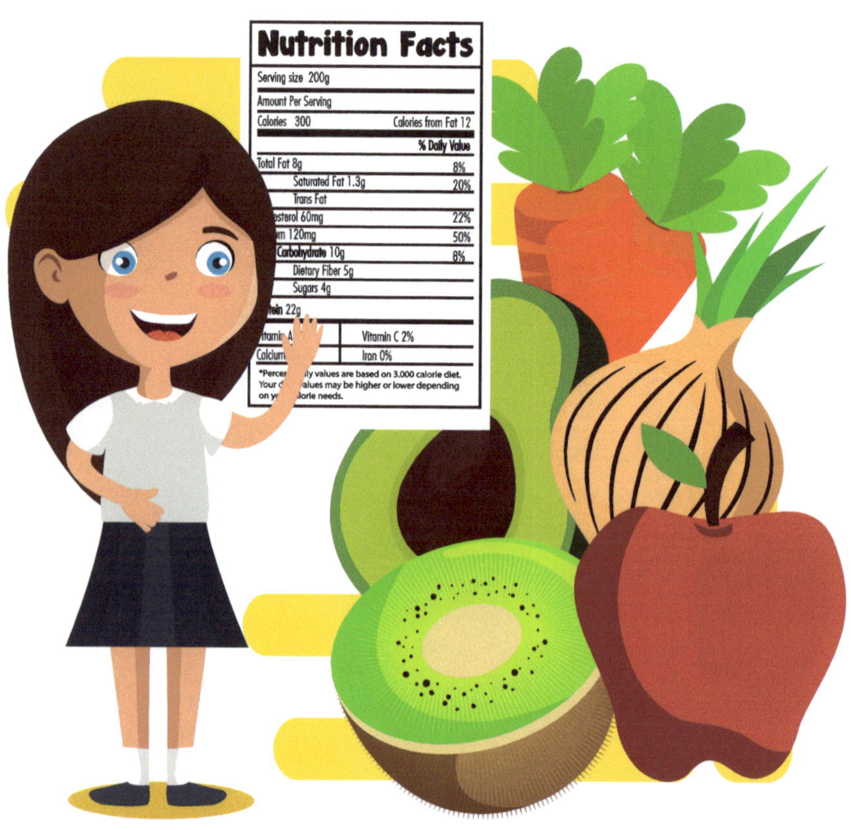

Over time, Ruhaani underwent a
transformation - her body
became strong, her spirit lively,
and her dreams achievable.

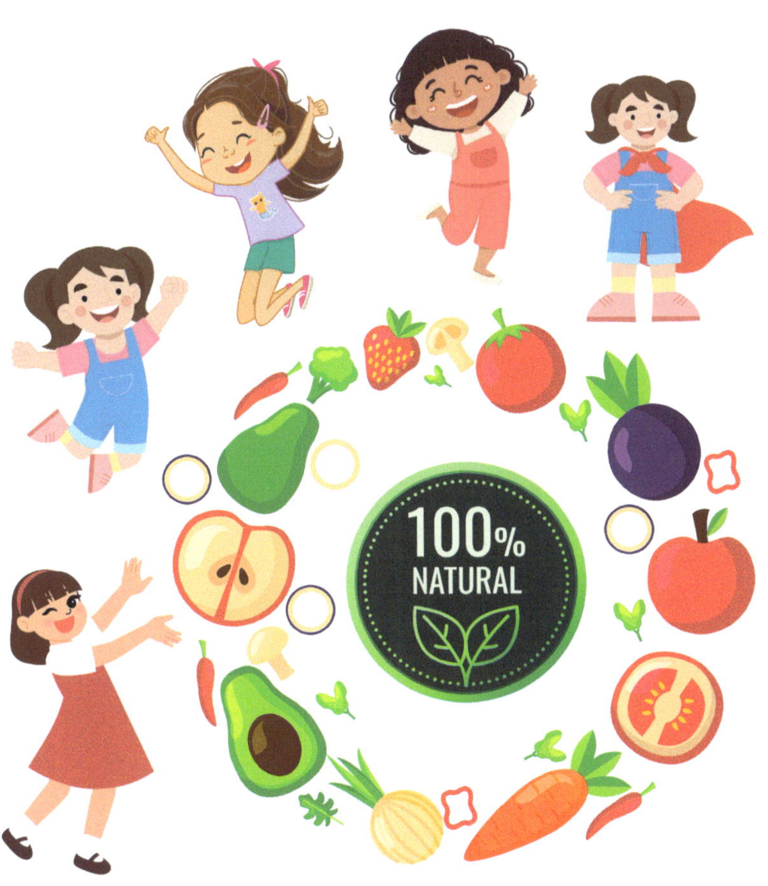

With a better understanding of
nutrition and a deep respect for the
influence of food, she set out on a
journey towards her ultimate goal -
the Olympics.

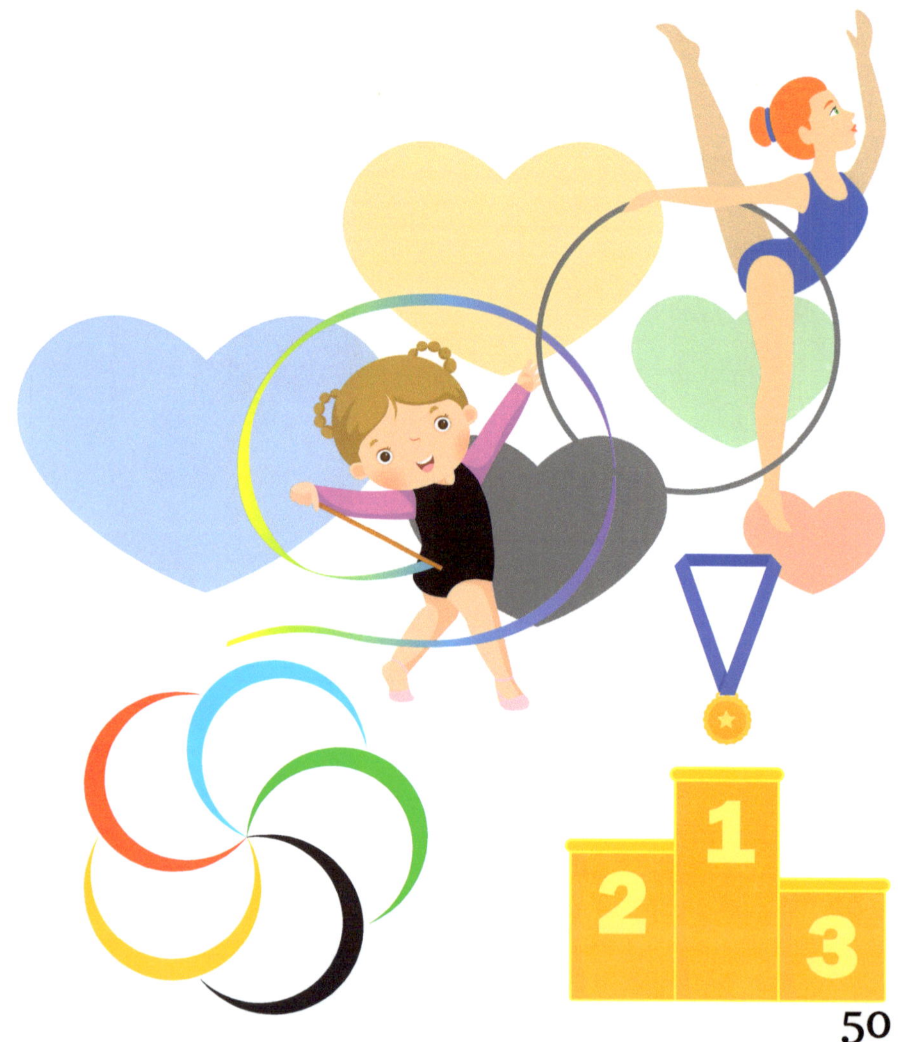